Learning Disabilities and Psychosocial Functioning

Learning Disabilities and Psychosocial Functioning

A Neuropsychological Perspective

BYRON P. ROURKE
DARREN R. FUERST
University of Windsor

THE GUILFORD PRESS
New York   London

© 1991 The Guilford Press
A Division of Guilford Publications, Inc.
72 Spring Street, New York, NY 10012

Printed in the United States of America

This book is printed on acid-free paper.

Last digit is print number: 9 8 7 6 5 4 3 2 1

Library of Congress Cataloging-in-Publication Data

Rourke, Byron P. (Byron Patrick), 1939–
    Learning disabilities and psychosocial functioning: a
neuropsychological perspective / Byron P. Rourke & Darren R. Fuerst.
        p. cm.
    Includes bibliographical references and index.
    ISBN 0-89862-767-2
    1. Learning disabled children—Mental health. 2. Social
interaction in children. 3. Neuropsychology. I. Fuerst, Darren R.
II. Title.
    [DNLM: 1. Adaptation, Psychological. 2. Learning Disorders.
3. Learning Disorders—in adulthood. WM 110 R862L]
RJ506.L4R67 1991
DNLM/DLC
for Library of Congress   91-16388
                                                              CIP

For Harry and Katy

Acknowledgments

We owe a debt of gratitude to many persons who assisted us in the production of this book. We are especially thankful to Joanna Hamilton and Sean B. Rourke, who were instrumental in assembling and analyzing the very large number of articles, chapters, and books that we found necessary to review. Marilyn Chedour read the entire text and, as usual, saved us from errors too embarrassing to mention. Finally, we wish to acknowledge the thoughtful efforts of the editorial staff of The Guilford Press; without their prodigious efforts, this work would never have seen the light of day.

BYRON P. ROURKE
DARREN R. FUERST

Contents

Chapter 1. Introduction and Overview 1

Chapter 2. Psychosocial Functioning of Children
with Learning Disabilities: Review of Hypotheses
1 and 2 4

Hypothesis 1: Socioemotional Disturbance Causes
Learning Disabilities, *4*
Hypothesis 2: Learning Disabilities Cause
Socioemotional Disturbance, *6*

Chapter 3. The Windsor Taxonomic Research 48

Study 1, *49*
Study 2, *50*
Study 3, *51*
Study 4, *52*
Study 5, *52*
Summary of Studies 1 through 5, *54*

Chapter 4. Psychosocial Functioning of Children
with Learning Disabilities: Review of Hypothesis 3,
and Conclusions 69

Hypothesis 3: Specific Patterns of Central Processing
Abilities and Deficits Cause Specific
Manifestations (Subtypes) of Learning Disabilities
and Specific Forms of Socioemotional
Disturbance, *69*
Conclusions, *85*

Chapter 5. Case Studies   90

     Introduction, *90*
     Case 1: John, *91*
     Case 2: Andrew, *101*
     Case 3: Chris, *109*
     Case 4: Jane, *117*
     Case 5: Carla, *131*
     Case 6: Mary, *139*
     Case 7: Michael, *146*
     Case 8: Roger, *155*
     Case 9: William, *165*

Chapter 6. Where We've Been and Where We're Going   175

     A Point of View, *175*
     General Clinical Implications, *176*
     Future Directions, *176*

References   179

Index   195

1

Introduction and Overview

The principal developmental demand for children in our society between the ages of 5 and 16 years is to learn in school. With the protracted "adolescence" spawned by the increasing complexities of our technological society, learning in school may, in fact, extend into the third and fourth decades of life. Even adults in the workplace, for whom school may be a fading memory, are often faced with demands to expand their knowledge and expertise. The accelerating pace of technological innovation and the economic upheavals characteristic of a modern industrial society require rapid adaptation by workers, ranging from periodic upgrading of skills and knowledge to complete retraining. It is ironic that while devices that can read, spell, and perform arithmetic are inexpensive and readily available to all, deficits in these basic skill areas can now have a greater impact on one's livelihood than at any time in the past.

Whether one is in school or not, employed or not, the capacity to benefit from experience and to fashion one's responses to meet the demands of such experience in an adaptive fashion (i.e., to learn) lies at the very core of what it is to be human. Hence, it should come as no surprise that disabilities in learning are thought to eventuate in much more than simple failure in school or failure to learn a job. Indeed, it is a commonly held notion that persons who experience significant difficulties in learning are most definitely susceptible to disorders in other areas of human functioning, such as the "emotional" and "social" dimensions of life. It is in this sense that some characterize learning disabilities (LD) as "life" or "lifetime" disabilities.

1

This book is our attempt to organize and present in a coherent fashion what is currently known about the psychosocial functioning of children with LD. In Chapters 2, 3, and 4, we examine research dealing with the relations between LD and socioemotional functioning—a subject that has generated considerable research activity over the past two decades. Although it is all but impossible to locate and read every published study related to this topic, we reviewed approximately 700 journal articles and research reviews in preparation for writing this book. Of this number, we felt that approximately 300 met minimal methodological standards and were worthy of more in-depth scrutiny. From this subset of approximately 300 publications we have selected studies that we feel are of particular value because they (1) contain findings that further our understanding of the psychosocial functioning of children with LD; (2) illustrate methodological innovations or, conversely, common methodological shortcomings; or (3) are of historical importance, having influenced later research efforts in this area.

The review itself is organized around three major hypotheses regarding the relations between socioemotional functioning and LD that have held sway from time to time over the past 20 years. The reviews of the evidence that relates to these hypotheses are followed by our characterization of the general and specific conclusions that can be arrived at on the basis of these reviews, and then by some clinical observations and generalizations that are felt to flow from the empirical evidence gathered to this point.

Of course, the principles regarding the socioemotional functioning of children with LD that we present in Chapters 2 through 4 are abstractions; persons, however, are not. At times it can be difficult to see how principles developed in the forced simplicity of the laboratory might help us to understand more fully the unique and complex difficulties faced by a particular child or adult experiencing learning problems. In Chapter 5, we present nine cases drawn from our files that illustrate the clinical application of the most important models and hypotheses developed in Chapters 2 through 4. We trust that the principles developed in these chapters, in combination with the real-world examples presented in Chapter 5, will prove useful to others working with persons with LD.

One final note is in order before we begin. Initially, we thought it might be possible to cover the entire age range in our review of the literature on this topic. However, we discovered quickly in our search for research in the area that few worthwhile investigations had been directed to the study of the relationships between psychosocial functioning and LD in adults. In retrospect, this should not have come as a surprise to us, since "learning disabilities" have been a subject of serious scientific scrutiny for only a relatively short period of time. Hence, there has been little opportunity to examine the long-term (adult) impact of childhood LD. Notable exceptions to this are the works of Spreen (1988) and Bruck (1987), and the recent volume of research by Johnson and Blalock (1987). These works are referred to in our review. However, the essentially exploratory nature of much of this research with adults and the unavailability of cross-validation attempts make it difficult to do much more than comment on what appear to be the very interesting hypotheses raised in this research with adults. Nevertheless, we do present two adult cases in Chapter 5, for the express purpose of demonstrating some of the long-term developmental dimensions of two different subtypes of LD.

With these observations as background, we turn now to our review of the literature.

2

Psychosocial Functioning of Children with Learning Disabilities: A Review of Hypotheses 1 and 2

In Chapters 2, 3, and 4, contemporary evidence that addresses two major hypotheses (Hypothesis 2 and Hypothesis 3 below) regarding the relationships between socioemotional functioning/disturbance and learning disabilities (LD) in children is reviewed. Where possible, we confine our remarks to relatively recent research (1980 or later), and include older studies only where they are of some historical significance or are especially germane to the immediate issues. In view of the large quantity of material to be reviewed, the potentially related topics of hyperactivity and attention deficit disorders are not addressed in these chapters; nor are treatment considerations discussed, except in conjunction with the case studies presented in Chapter 5.

HYPOTHESIS 1: Socioemotional Disturbance Causes Learning Disabilities

Before we deal with the two hypotheses that are of particular concern to us, another, widely held position (Hypothesis 1) should be outlined and discussed: specifically, the notion that socioemotional disturbance causes LD. In this view, learning problems that children face in school and elsewhere are thought to constitute one reflection of systematic disturbances in socioemotional functioning (e.g., unresolved psychic conflicts). The evidence for this assertion comes from a variety of sources; some are empirical (e.g., Colbert, Newman, Ney, & Young, 1982), but most are "clinical" in nature (e.g., Brumback & Staton, 1983; Ehrlich, 1983). For example, many observers whose professional work brings them into contact with youngsters who are experiencing problems in academic achievement have noted that a significant proportion of these children suffer from one or more difficulties of a socioemotional sort—for example, personality conflicts with their teachers that render learning in the classroom difficult, if not impossible; strain associated with difficulties in meeting the (exaggerated) perceived demands of their parents and teachers; extreme psychic conflicts that render them almost incapable of benefiting from ordinary scholastic instruction; "inappropriate" motivation for academic success and social expectancies at variance with those of the school; major psychiatric disorders, such as depression, that remain undiagnosed and/or untreated (Rourke, Bakker, Fisk, & Strang, 1983; Rourke, Fisk, & Strang, 1986). These examples illustrate the following: that social conflict between teacher and student should be kept to a minimum if academic learning is to proceed apace; that unrealistic ego ideals can, and usually do, have a profound negative impact on performance; that significant intrapsychic conflicts or psychiatric disorders, no matter how generated and maintained, can have a significant impact on academic performance; and that the school is largely a middle-class institution that requires at least the temporary adoption of its standards (in North America, largely those of the Protestant ethic) for success in its programs.

These few examples should serve to illustrate the enormous number of complex sets of interactions that can serve to limit significantly the academic progress of untold numbers of students. In all of these instances, the socioemotional "problem" antedates the difficulty in learning; this is so even in the first example cited above. Furthermore, it is assumed that, were the socioemotional problem to be resolved, satisfactory academic performance would ensue. Thus, solving the student–teacher personality conflict, bringing ego ideals more closely into tune with reality, rectifying the intrapsychic conflict or psychiatric disorder, and leading the student to adopt a motivational posture and social expectancy set that are more in line with those of the school would be expected to lead eventually to satisfactory academic progress. The recent work of Rothstein, Benjamin, Crosby, and Eisenstadt (1988) contains excellent examples of the manner in which primary socioemotional disturbance can lead to difficulties in learning. The interested reader may also wish to consult Rourke, Fisk, and Strang (1986, pp. 177–182) for a discussion and case example of this cause–effect relationship.

This having been said, it is also necessary to point out that these matters really have to do with academic and other learning difficulties that are not usually included under the rubric of "learning disability." The latter term is commonly reserved for persons whose significant problems in learning are *not* a result of primary emotional disturbance (or mental retardation, primary sensory handicap, inadequate instruction, inappropriate motivation, or cultural/linguistic deprivation—the "exclusionary" criteria embodied in most definitions of LD). Thus, although interesting in and of themselves, and of obvious importance for the total understanding and treatment of children's problems in learning, these factors are not properly considered within the context of socioemotional correlates of LD. Hence, the remainder of this review is devoted to those considerations that fall quite precisely within the latter domain.

HYPOTHESIS 2: Learning Disabilities
Cause Socioemotional Disturbance

The first major hypothesis of interest within the present context is one that, like Hypothesis 1, proposes a causal link between learning difficulties and socioemotional disturbance (Rourke & Fisk, 1981). The differences in this instance are that (1) "learning disability," as commonly defined (Rourke, 1975), is the focus of interest; and (2) the causal relationship is reversed—that is, it is proposed that LD lead to disrupted or aberrant psychosocial functioning. This general proposition has a very compelling, tacit appeal for most clinicians; it concretizes a view that is widely held and that has become almost a cornerstone of clinical lore in this area.

The reasons for the *prima facie* appeal of this view are numerous. For example, it appears to make good clinical sense to maintain that a youngster with LD whose learning problems persist throughout the elementary school years will be the unwilling (and perhaps unwitting) butt of criticism and negative evaluations by parents, teachers, and age-mates; that these criticisms will serve to render the learning-disabled child more anxious and less self-assured in learning situations; that a vicious circle will develop that increasingly hampers academic success and encourages progressively debilitating degrees of anxiety (i.e., learning failure results in increased anxiety, which results in feelings of inferiority, which results in additional learning failure, etc.); and that this sort of undesirable situation is virtually inevitable and would be expected to increase in severity as the child fails to make advances in learning.

Research in support of this position has focused on the emotional, social, and behavioral functioning of children with LD, with particular regard to their interpersonal environment. In our review of research dealing with this hypothesis, we examine current research relevant to, or advanced in support of, variants of this general hypothesis. Four specific areas of investigation are scrutinized: (1) patterns of general psychosocial functioning and pathology; (2) social status with respect to peers and teachers; (3) self-concept/self-esteem and attributions; and (4) social competence. Methodological problems with a good deal of this research are also briefly discussed.

Psychosocial Functioning and Pathology

The various techniques that have been used to assess general aspects of psychosocial functioning and psychopathology in children with LD are as diverse as are those applied to any other subgroup of children with developmental disabilities. Many classification schemes have been used to categorize and summarize the results of studies in this area, and, as in other areas of LD literature, there is no consensus regarding the "best" scheme. In this exposition, we examine studies utilizing observation of classroom behavior, checklists/rating scales, personality inventories, and longitudinal outcomes. Note that we do not examine the specific *methodological* pros and cons of these various approaches (see, e.g., Schumaker &

Hazel, 1984, for this information), and that we also assume that readers are familiar with the measurement methods and instruments used in the studies reviewed below (see, e.g., Barkley, 1988, for detailed descriptions). Our evaluations of these findings are high-lighted at the end of each section.

Observation of Classroom Behavior

Whereas some investigators have relied on psychometric instru-ments to assess psychosocial functioning of children with LD (see below), others have adapted behavior analysis procedures, and have introduced direct observation methods into the classroom. The uti-lization of this group of techniques seems to have become somewhat less popular in recent years, despite evidence suggesting that mea-sures of classroom behavior may be useful for predicting academic achievement in normal children (McKinney, Mason, Perkerson, & Clifford, 1975). For a detailed review of such studies prior to 1978, see Hoge and Luce (1979). Note that most direct observation studies included in this review (such as those of Bryan or McKinney and colleagues) are reviewed in other sections, where they have particu-lar relevance to the topic under consideration. Only two representa-tive studies are examined in this section.

In an early study, Richey and McKinney (1978) contrasted the behavior of 15 third- and fourth-grade male students with LD (identi-fied in a previous study) with a matched sample of normally achiev-ing students from the same classrooms. Richey and McKinney used two observers per matched subject pair (with data collected across a 3-day period) on 12 general categories of behavior (covering task-oriented, social, and affective dimensions), at 10-second intervals over a 10-minute period (i.e., 180 instances of observation per subject). Overall, the children with LD differed from normal children on only one dimension, distractibility. The children with LD showed no evidence of the negative behaviors often ascribed to them, such as con-duct problems, hyperactivity, or passivity and dependency. Similar results regarding task-oriented behavior/distractibility have been re-ported in subsequent studies (e.g., Feagans & McKinney, 1981; McKinney & Speece, 1983; Tarver & Hallahan, 1974).

More recently, Sprafkin and Gadow (1987) compared the observed behaviors of 26 male students with LD (identified by the school system) and 27 male students with emotional disturbance (ED) between the ages of 5 and 9 years. Two observers collected data on each subject across a 3-day period, on five general categories of behavior (physical and nonphysical aggression, noncompliance, immature and socially inappropriate behaviors), at 30-second intervals over a 6-minute period, in three different settings (classroom, lunch, and recess). Overall, the results were thought to demonstrate that the children with ED demonstrated much more noncompliant and aggressive behavior than did the children with LD. Sprafkin and Gadow (1987) concluded that, contrary to results that would be expected in terms of Hypothesis 2, children with LD and children with ED differ significantly on important, intervention-relevant behaviors. In a word, children with LD differ significantly from children with ED in terms of behaviors that are used to categorize the children with ED as suffering from socioemotional disturbance.

Checklists/Rating Scales

In a seminal investigation in this area, McCarthy and Paraskevopoulos (1969) compared the Behavior Problem Checklist (BPC; Quay & Peterson, 1975) scores of 36 students with LD (unspecified selection criteria), 100 students with ED, and 41 normal students, as rated by their teachers. The raw scores were transformed to scores on three factors identified in previous research (viz., Unsocialized Aggression, Immaturity–Inadequacy, and Personality Problem). In general, the children with ED were rated worst; normal children, best; and children with LD at levels intermediate to the other two groups. The main behavior problem of both children with LD and children with ED was conduct problem behavior (disruptiveness, problems with attention, fighting, etc.). In the learning-disabled group, problems of immaturity–inadequacy and neurotic behavior were of about equal importance; however, in the emotionally disturbed group, the latter behaviors were of less importance. McCarthy and Paraskevopoulos (1969) concluded that although children with LD and children with ED share some behavioral characteristics that distinguish them from normal children, these two groups also demonstrate some quite unique features.

Gajar (1979) reported somewhat different results when she compared the BPC ratings of 135 children with LD (identified by unspecified means), 122 children with ED, and 121 educable mentally retarded children. In this study, instead of calculating factor scores (as did McCarthy & Paraskevopoulos, 1969), the investigator summed ratings on the items for each factor and transformed them into a percentage of total items for that factor (a somewhat unusual procedure). Gajar found that the emotionally disturbed group scored significantly worse than the learning-disabled or educable mentally retarded groups on the Conduct Disorder and Personality Problem factors, and worse than the educable mentally retarded group on the Immaturity–Inadequacy dimension. This would suggest that, as in the previous study, there are some similarities, but also some very noteworthy differences, between children with ED and children with LD.

A study by Richmond and Blagg (1985) generated results even more divergent from those of McCarthy and Paraskevopoulos (1969). In this investigation, school-identified groups of learning-disabled, behavior-disordered, educable mentally retarded, and normal children were compared on four dimensions of the BPC. Overall, the normal, learning-disabled, and educable mentally retarded groups were indistinguishable. Only the behavior-disordered group scored significantly worse on BPC dimensions. Abelson and Mutsch (1985) have reported similar results using a different rating scale; that is, they found no differences in adaptive behavior between children with LD and children with mild mental retardation.

Cullinan, Epstein, and colleagues have published a number of studies comparing the BPC scores of learning-disabled and other subgroups of children. For example, Cullinan, Epstein, and Lloyd (1981) compared the BPC teacher ratings of 50 learning-disabled (identified by the school system) and 50 normal students, ranging from 6 to 18 years of age, matched for age and sex (25 males and 25 females in each group). Sums of mild and severe ratings on items were used to derive scores on three dimensions of the BPC (Conduct Disorder, Personality Problem, and Inadequacy–Immaturity). Overall, the students with LD demonstrated more behavior problems than did normal students. Further analyses revealed that the children with LD differed from the normal children only on the Personality Problem dimension. Although, overall, boys tended to show more behavior problems than did girls, there were no significant sex differences on any of the specific dimensions. Cullinan et al. (1981) concluded that children with LD show socioemotional differences from normal children in areas of anxiety, self-confidence, withdrawal, depression, and similar behaviors, as measured by the Personality Problem dimension of the BPC.

Epstein and Cullinan (1984) attempted to extend these findings by comparing the BPC scores of 13 age-matched quartets of normal, learning-disabled, educable mentally retarded, and behavior-disordered (identification techniques unspecified) male high school students. In this study, scores on four dimensions of the BPC (Conduct Disorder, Personality Problem, Inadequacy–Immaturity, and Socialized Delinquency) were calculated in the same manner used by Cullinan et al. (1981). The investigators found that the BPC could discriminate the normal students from all other groups on the Personality Problem and Conduct Disorder dimensions. The behavior-disordered group scored worse than all other groups on all dimensions. The learning-disabled group performed much like the educable mentally retarded group (i.e., midway between the normal and behavior-disordered groups), with the exception that the educable mentally retarded group showed higher Inadequacy–Immaturity scores. Epstein and Cullinan (1984) argued that, considering the results of previous research (Cullinan, Epstein, & Dembinski, 1979; Cullinan et al., 1981), it would appear that as children with LD become older, teachers tend to see them as becoming somewhat worse in terms of psychosocial functioning. This view was based on the finding that the older children with LD in the study scored higher than did normal children on both the Conduct Disorder and Personality Problem dimensions, rather than just on the latter dimension, as was found in the Cullinan et al. (1981) study.

Noting that most studies of learning-disabled and behavior-disordered students have used a preponderance of male subjects, Cullinan, Schultz, Epstein, and Luebke (1984) formed 45 age-matched quartets of normal, learning-disabled, educable mentally retarded, and behavior-disordered females between the ages of 12 and 16 years; they then compared them on four BPC dimensions, calculated in the same manner used in Epstein and Cullinan (1984).

The results were similar to those found by Epstein and Cullinan (1984). Behavior-disordered subjects scored more highly on the Conduct Disorder, Inadequacy–Immaturity, and Socialized Delinquency dimensions than did the other groups. The educable mentally retarded children obtained scores equivalent to those of normal subjects on all dimensions. The learning-disabled and behavior-disordered girls scored at comparable levels on the Personality Problem dimension, with both showing significantly more problems than did the normal subjects. Cullinan et al. (1984) concluded that learning-disabled (and behavior-disordered) girls demonstrate psychosocial problems that are quite similar to those found in learning-disabled (and behavior-disordered) boys.

In a subsequent study by Epstein, Cullinan, and Bursuck (1985), a somewhat different procedure was used to analyze BPC scores. In this study, the investigators collected BPC ratings on relatively large samples of younger (aged 6–11 years) and older (aged 12–18 years) male and female learning-disabled and normal (school-identified) students. Rather than calculating scores on the major BPC dimensions, as was done in previous studies, the investigators determined the prevalence of each BPC item within each of the subgroups (i.e., the percentage of the total subgroup for which an item was checked). Overall, the students with LD were rated as being substantially more deviant than were the normal subjects. Specifically, students with LD showed more attentional problems, as well as more social and emotional coping problems (such as anxiety); males with LD also showed more aggressive conduct problems. The aggressive problem behaviors noted typically involved classroom disruption rather than truly delinquent behaviors (such as stealing). Students with LD also showed a much higher incidence of mild motor impairments (from two to five times the incidence in normal children for learning-disabled boys and girls, respectively). Within the learning-disabled group, the incidence of attention problems tended to decrease with age. The learning-disabled girls tended to show more "internalized" problems at later ages, whereas learning-disabled boys tended to become more rebellious and "externalized."

Research with other behavior rating scales and checklists has provided essentially similar results. For example, Cohen and Hynd (1986) and Margalit (1989) have reported findings similar to those of

McCarthy and Paraskevopoulos (1969), using the Conners Teacher Rating Scale (Conners, 1969, 1973); that is, they have found that children with LD and children with behavior problems demonstrate rather different patterns of psychosocial functioning. Harris, King, Reifler, and Rosenberg (1984) compared 30 male 6- to 12-year-old children with LD (State-identified) to 30 matched children with ED on teacher-completed Child Behavior Checklist (CBCL; Achenbach, 1978; Achenbach & Edelbrock, 1979, 1981, 1983) scores. Overall, the emotionally disturbed boys showed much more behavior disturbance than did the learning-disabled boys. However, about 50% of the learning-disabled boys had CBCL scores falling within the "clinical" range, and within this subgroup of students with LD a wide range of pathology was observed (aggressive behavior was relatively common). McConaughy and Ritter (1986) collected parent-completed CBCL scores for 123 male 6- to 11-year-olds with LD (identified by individual psychoeducational assessment). As compared to CBCL norms, the children with LD exhibited lower social competence and more behavior problems at rates of clinical significance for both the internalizing and externalizing variety. However, McConaughy and Ritter (1986) noted that relatively few of the children exhibited a delinquent profile.

A Note on Delinquent Behavior

At this point it is well to examine briefly the potential link between LD and delinquent/antisocial behavior. The reader is referred to a recent review by Larson (1988) for a more detailed examination of this issue. A number of studies have indicated that there is a marked coincidence of learning problems and delinquent/antisocial behavior. For example, Sturge (1982) found that in a sample of 1,689 children aged 10, 11% exhibited evidence of reading retardation, and 17% exhibited antisocial behavior. There was an overlap of 3.6% between these two categories (i.e., children exhibiting both reading retardation and antisocial behavior). This percentage is small, but it is also somewhat greater than that which would be expected by chance alone (i.e., 2.2%). In Larson's (1988) review in which LD and delinquency was investigated, the co-occurrence of the two varied between 26% and 73%.

Unfortunately, methodological problems are rampant in, if not virtually endemic to, this area of research. A study by Wilgosh and Paitich (1982) is an excellent example of this point. They examined 99 adjudicated delinquents, and found that more than 60% of the subjects were "learning-disabled." However, they failed to assess level of psychometric intelligence adequately; they used only the Raven's Progressive Matrices test (Raven, 1960) and the Vocabulary subtest of the Wechsler Intelligence Scale for Children (WISC; Wechsler, 1949). They also failed to screen for educational and cultural deprivation, perceptual and speech anomalies, primary psychopathology, and a number of other very important dimensions of developmental disabilities. Furthermore, their "diagnosis" of "LD" was essentially made solely on the basis of discrepancies between Wide Range Achievement Test (WRAT; Jastak & Jastak, 1965) subtest scores and grade placement. In view of these limitations, the results of the Wilgosh and Paitich (1982) study suggest, at most, that a high proportion of adjudicated delinquents show evidence of academic underachievement.

The results of most studies described in this and other sections of our review indicate that the vast majority of children with LD do not demonstrate truly antisocial or delinquent behavior. As Sturge (1982) has pointed out, there is no simple association between LD and antisocial/delinquent behavior (i.e., the apparent relationship may be an artifact), and associated factors, such as cultural differences, low socioeconomic status (SES), inadequate family environment, antisocial peers, and other disadvantageous influences, must be properly assessed before valid conclusions can be drawn regarding the proposed linkage. The interested reader is referred to studies by Bryan, Werner, and Pearl (1982), and Schumaker, Hazel, Sherman, and Sheldon (1982) for interesting results regarding conformity and peer influence in this context.

Personality Inventories

As Goh, Cody, and Dollinger (1984) have pointed out, personality assessment of children with LD by means of "objective" inventories has been relatively rare, perhaps due to the paucity of suitable instruments. One personality inventory that has been employed rather extensively in empirical studies in this area is the Personality Inventory for Children (PIC; Wirt, Lachar, Klinedinst, & Seat, 1977, 1984). The PIC is an interesting research tool in that it is relatively convenient to administer and score, provides good coverage of various behavioral domains, has acceptable norms, and has actuarial interpretive guidelines (see Wirt et al., 1977, 1984, for details).

Harrington and Marks (1985) noted that commonly used procedures for assessing psychosocial adaptation in diagnostic contexts may require substantial professional resources. They noted the convenience and other laudable aspects of the PIC, and wondered whether the Adjustment scale (a measure of general psychosocial functioning) could serve as a screening instrument in psychoeducational assessment. To this end, they compared the Adjustment scale scores of 11 normal, 14 learning-disabled, and 10 behavior-disordered children in grades 1 to 6. The results showed that the Adjustment scores of the behavior-disordered children were significantly higher (i.e., suggesting greater pathology) than were those of both the normal and learning-disabled subjects. Although the learning-disabled subjects showed a mean Adjustment score within the clinical range (72 T), this was not significantly higher than that of the normal children (60 T). Although Harrington and Marks (1985) were suitably cautious in interpreting their results, they failed to note that the Adjustment scores of the learning-disabled subjects also showed a substantial degree of variability (a standard deviation of about 23 T-score points), suggesting that some of these children had distinctly pathological elevations on this scale.

A study carried out by Forbes (1987) confirms the finding that children with LD may exhibit clinically significant elevations of the PIC Adjustment scale. When the Adjustment scores of 100 children (6 to 12 years of age) referred to a private clinic were examined, 46% of children with scores greater than 84 T had a diagnosis of LD (made by the school system), versus 12% of children with scores below 84 T. This was thought to suggest some association between LD and disordered psychosocial functioning.

Other researchers have examined the full complement of PIC scores, in an attempt to determine whether PIC profiles can discriminate LD from other diagnostic categories. For example, Goh et al. (1984) contrasted the PIC profiles of 30 learning-disabled children (diagnosed by an "interdisciplinary team") and 30 behavior-disordered children, with a mean age of about 9 years. The results showed that, overall, the PIC profiles of the children with LD were within roughly normal limits, whereas the profiles of behavior-disordered children showed significant elevations on a number of scales. Using a profile classification system developed by DeHorn, Lachar, and Gdowski (1979), Goh et al. (1984) found that about 27% of subjects with LD had normal PIC profiles, 37% had profiles indicative of respondent concerns over cognitive development, and about 20% had profiles characterized by concern with both cognitive development and internalized psychopathology. Overall, only 36% of subjects with LD had PIC profiles indicative of psychopathology, versus 87% of such profiles for the behavior-disordered subjects. Results roughly consistent with those of Goh et al. (1984) have also been reported by Forbes (1987).

Longitudinal Studies

Common to Hypothesis 2 approaches is the notion that the negative consequences of LD, in some manner, distort the development of psychosocial adaptation over time. It is often argued that as children with LD grow older, their socioemotional difficulties should worsen. Even if academically related frustration and failure become less important as children move toward adulthood, the adaptive demands that are commensurate with advancing age do not lessen. Indeed, one could reasonably expect that these demands probably become more complex, with consequent negative impact on psychosocial functioning for those who do not achieve at developmentally appropriate levels. For example, Capute and Accardo (1980) have maintained that the typical adolescent with LD is likely to become "an illiterate, unemployable teenage dropout, addict, and potential suicide" (p. 298).

Some researchers have followed children with LD for extended periods of time to determine whether, indeed, the long-term prospects for these children are poor. With respect to psychosocial functioning, early studies produced equivocal results (see Horn, O'Donnell, & Vitulano, 1983, for a review of research prior to 1980, and a discussion of methodological issues). Specifically, these studies provided evidence for both poor (Cerny, 1976; Werner & Smith, 1979) and adequate (Abott & Frank, 1975; Edgington, 1975) psychosocial outcomes for persons with LD. A representative sample of the results of studies in this area follows.

Fafard and Haubrich (1981) conducted a follow-up study of 21 young adults (aged 16 to 23 years) with LD (diagnosis based on standardized testing), at anywhere from 10 to 19 years after initial contact with the investigators' institution. An interview, consisting of 20 questions covering academic, vocational, and social adjustment, was administered to subjects and their parents. In general, the majority of subjects had finished high school, found employment, and had adequate psychosocial adaptation. A small number of parents did express concern about their children's ability to make friends, and some subjects did appear to be dependent on family members for social activities (this was more so, perhaps, for females). The greatest difficulties for these children (now adults) appeared to be in the area of career/vocational counseling and assistance. Psychosocial outcomes seemed to be relatively benign (i.e., there was no significant degree of psychopathology reported).

Levin, Zigmond, and Birch (1985) carried out a 4-year follow-up study of 34 children with LD, identified as such by the school system when in ninth grade (most had already been recognized or diagnosed as learning-disabled by age 9). Four years later, about 30% of the participating students (i.e., 11 subjects) had left school, and most of those remaining in school were still receiving special education. Of those dropouts who participated in the study, about 60% (7 of 11 students) had been asked to leave school because of behavior problems. Although only 2 of 11 (18%) dropouts were employed, 8 of 11 (73%) were enroled in alternative (general equivalency diploma, or GED) or vocational programs. Self-concept scores (discussed in detail below), as measured by a standard instrument, were within normal limits initially (in the ninth grade) and showed positive increases at follow-up. Considering that this was a clearly disadvantaged sample at the commencement of the study (i.e., 4 years before follow-up), and that at follow-up most had either dropped out of school or were still receiving special education, the psychosocial outcome—to the limited extent that it was addressed in this study—would appear, once again, to be relatively good.

Jorm, Share, Matthews, and Maclean (1986) assessed 543 children entering kindergarten on psychosocial measures, and again at 2 and 3 years after entering school. At the end of the study, children were administered various cognitive and reading tests, and classified as either normal, "specific retarded readers" (readers whose achievement was below predictions based on age and cognitive measures), or "backward readers" (underachieving readers not meeting the criterion for specific retarded readers). The results were thought to demonstrate that backward (underachieving) readers had behavioral problems, primarily in the domain of attention deficits and hyperactivity, at the time they entered school; normal and specific retarded readers did not differ on these measures. Jorm et al. (1986) speculated, for the backward readers, that either behavioral problems were causing the reading problems or some common factor was causing both the reading and emotional problems. Indeed, the specific retarded readers (i.e., those whom many would label as learning-disabled) showed no psychosocial disturbance either at school entry or after their reading problems had become manifest.

McGee, Williams, Share, Anderson, and Silva (1986) performed a similar study, taking psychosocial ratings from teachers and parents for children at 5, 7, 9, and 11 years of age. The children selected for investigation were 18 boys with specific reading retardation (reading substantially below prediction based on Wechsler Intelligence Scale for Children—Revised [WISC-R; Wechsler, 1974] Performance IQ [PIQ] score; i.e., reading-disabled), 22 boys with general reading backwardness (reading lower than age expectations, but not substantially below predicted level based on PIQ), and a comparison group of 436 other boys meeting neither of these criteria. The results were thought to demonstrate that both groups of children with reading difficulties manifested problem behaviors at school entry (mainly of aggressive and hyperactive types), and that these problems tended to become somewhat worse over time (peaking at about age 9, but continuing at relatively high levels at age 11) especially for the reading-disabled boys. At age 11, 57% of the reading disabled boys met *Diagnostic and Statistical Manual of Mental Disorders*, third edition (DSM-III) diagnostic criteria for psychiatric disorder (mainly Attention Deficit Disorder, Conduct Disorder, and/or Oppositional Defiant Disorder), as did 47% of the children with general reading backwardness; this contrasted with 18% of the comparison group so classified. In contrast to Jorm et al. (1986), McGee et al. (1986) concluded that reading-disabled children are about three times as likely to evidence psychopathology as are normal children, and that the problem behaviors of these children worsen with age. However, it should be noted that the children with general reading backwardness in this study showed similar socio-emotional disturbance, and, as problem behaviors were already present on entry to school, reading difficulties per se could not be directly causing problems in psychosocial functioning. Results similar to these with non-learning-disabled children have been reported by Kohn and Rosman (1974).

Finally, Spreen and colleagues have carried out longitudinal studies of children with LD over a time span of more than 15 years. The results of this project are summarized in Spreen (1988). Given the wealth of published material that has been generated from this research, the following synopsis has been derived from that source. We recommend that interested readers refer to Spreen (1988) for detailed information and relevant citations.

In the first phase of the research documented in Spreen (1988), 203 children with LD (identified as such by means of standardized measures and exclusionary criteria) and their parents were interviewed about 9 years after their first contact with the investigators. A matched sample of 52 children was selected as a control group. In addition to a structured interview, behavior rating scales and a personality inventory were administered. The results at the first follow-up were not encouraging: The learning-disabled subjects showed evidence of greater socioemotional disturbance and antisocial behavior than did the controls. There was, however, no difference in the number of contacts with the police or offenses committed by learning-disabled or control subjects, and there were no differences in the use of alcohol or illegal drugs. Thus, overall, there was no evidence of greater delinquency in the learning-disabled group.

In the second phase of the research program, subjects were again assessed about 6 years after the first phase. By then, most subjects were in their mid-20s. The results were comparable to those found in the first phase. There was no evidence of greater delinquency or drug use in the learning-disabled group. However, the subjects with LD did experience greater psychosocial disturbance.

On the Minnesota Multiphasic Personality Inventory (MMPI), the learning-disabled females tended to have profiles suggestive of low self-confidence, brooding, social alienation, and depression; males tended to show evidence of autistic behavior and disruptive thought. Spreen (1988) concluded that, overall, the long-term psychosocial outcome for children with LD is relatively poor. However, he cautioned that variability in outcomes among the subjects was substantial. Some of the learning-disabled subjects were productive, well-adjusted members of the community, whereas others were found in group homes, prisons, or institutions.

Summary

Although the results of studies employing classroom observations, checklists/rating scales, personality inventories, and longitudinal methods are often contradictory, it would appear that as a group, children with LD are at somewhat greater risk for aberrant psychosocial development or psychopathology. However, it is also clear that not all children with LD fare poorly in these respects: The range of psychosocial outcomes is probably as great as that seen in normal children (i.e., some do very well, some do moderately well, some do poorly, etc.). On average, children with LD may fare worse than their normal peers, but reliable estimates of the incidence of various degrees and types of disordered psychosocial adaptation have not emerged from the literature. Considering the studies reviewed above, we must conclude that a simple and clear causal link between LD and psychopathology has not been demonstrated.

Social Status

The extent to which children with LD are accepted, rejected, or ignored by peers and teachers has been a lively area of investigation for the last 15 years or so. There appear to be two main reasons for this interest. First, the social status of children with LD may provide a general marker of socioemotional functioning, as it seems logical to assume that children with psychosocial deficits or frank psychopathology will have difficulty interacting with and gaining the acceptance of peers and teachers. Second, social status may interact with psychosocial functioning in a bidirectional manner: That is, low social status may adversely affect psychosocial functioning, which in turn may affect social status, and so on. However, some researchers (e.g., Asher, 1983) have proposed purely unidirectional as opposed to interactional models. The volume of studies in this area precludes a completely detailed review within the present context. For studies prior to the mid-1980s, the reader is referred to two comprehensive and cogent reviews by Dudley-Marling and Edmiaston (1985) and Wiener (1987). For our present purposes, studies of historical interest and more recent investigations are discussed in this section, which is divided in terms of the techniques typically employed in such studies.

Nomination Techniques

Perhaps the most often cited study of social status of children with LD is an investigation by Bryan (1974b). In this study, the sociometric status of 84 learning-disabled students (identified by school authorities) in grades 3, 4, and 5 was contrasted with the status of normal subjects matched on sex, race, and classroom. A "nomination" technique, in which the children in a classroom are asked to identify other children with various positive and negative social characteristics (e.g., best friend, most attractive, most anxious), was employed. Bryan examined the intercorrelations of the nomination items, and identified two major independent dimensions of status: social acceptance and social rejection. Overall, the learning-disabled students received fewer acceptance nominations and more rejection nominations than did control students. On the dimension of rejection nominations, there was also a statistically significant sex $\times$ group (learning-disabled vs. control) interaction. Bryan (1974b) interpreted this interaction as a much greater rejection of female students with LD relative to other subgroups. However, Dudley-Marling and Edmiaston (1985) have pointed out that this conclusion is, in fact, a misinterpretation of the interaction effect. Be that as it may, the findings of the Bryan (1974b) investigation were essentially replicated in subsequent studies by the same author (Bryan, 1976; Bryan & Bryan, 1978).

Other researchers using similar techniques have found essentially the same results as did Bryan (1974b). For example, Scranton and Ryckman (1979) compared peer nominations of 42 primary students with LD (identified using exclusionary criteria) with control subjects matched by homeroom. The investigators found that, as in the Bryan (1974b, 1976) studies, students with LD received fewer positive nominations and more negative nominations than did control subjects. Female students with LD also appeared to be more rejected relative to other subgroups, and there were, in fact, no significant differences between normal and learning-disabled males on either positive or negative items. It should be pointed out, however, that subsequent studies either have not reported or have not found gender differences in social status (Wiener, 1987; see, e.g., Shirer, Wiener, & Harris, 1988).

One final note regarding the Scranton and Ryckman investigation is in order: In this study, the school used an "open concept" system in which students moved about frequently. The investigators maintained that this would control for the potential stigma of attending special education classes. However, they did not carry out any empirical tests of this assertion. Indeed, recent research by Stephens, Wiener, and Harris (1988) has shown that degree of integration into the regular classroom is positively related to social status (i.e., greater integration is related to higher social status).

Siperstein, Bopp, and Bak (1978) compared peer nominations of 22 students with LD (identified by the school system) to those of 155 normal classmates. The authors elicited nominations in three major domains (academic ability, athletic ability, and physical attractiveness) plus general acceptance ("Whom do you like the best?"). The results showed that, overall, learning-disabled students were significantly less popular than were their normal peers. However, there were no differences in the domains of athletic ability or physical attractiveness. Also, learning-disabled students were no more likely to be "isolates" (i.e., not nominated as a friend) than were normal students. Students with LD were, however, underrepresented in the "star" category (i.e., nominated by a high proportion of peers). Siperstein et al. (1978) argued that children with LD may be socially hampered, but are not necessarily rejected, perhaps because of their strengths in nonacademic areas such as athletics.

A more recent study using the nomination technique has been reported by Landau, Milich, and McFarland (1987). This investigation is of interest because of the relative sophistication of its design. Landau et al. (1987) wondered whether the social status difficulties of children with LD that were identified in previous studies were due to difficulties of a subgroup of these children, rather than being characteristic of all children with LD. It employed 65 male third- to sixth-grade learning-disabled students (identified by the school system plus exclusionary criteria) and their normally achieving male classmates. The students with LD were subdivided on the basis of WISC-R Verbal IQ (VIQ)–PIQ discrepancy (viz., VIQ = PIQ within 8 points, VIQ > PIQ by at least 15 points, or VIQ < PIQ by at least 15 points). (The general rationale for such an approach is discussed in detail in Chapter 4 of this book.) The results confirmed that not all male children with LD experience problems in social status. In general, the VIQ > PIQ children showed no significant differences in positive or negative peer evaluations, relative to normally achieving classmates. In contrast, the VIQ = PIQ children were less popular and more likely to be rejected than normal children. The VIQ < PIQ subjects were less popular than normal children, and were also nominated as being more socially withdrawn.

Rating Scales

The second method used to assess social status is that of rating scales. In this technique, subjects are presented with a list of peers and are asked to rate them on various attributes (such as attraction, aggression, like–dislike, and so on). Theoretically, rating scales may provide more detailed information about social status than do nomination measures: Each child is rated by all classmates, and, as names of all classmates are provided, children cannot inadvertently overlook certain peers (Sainato, Zigmond, & Strain, 1983). Also, there is clearly a difference between not being nominated as "best friend" or "best athlete" and not being accepted by peers.

In two of the earliest studies employing peer rating, Bruininks (1978a, 1978b) contrasted the peer-rated social status of elementary school students with LD (identified by the school system) with that of normally achieving peers. In the first study, Bruininks (1978a) found that, overall, learning-disabled students received lower ratings relative to total class ratings, but only learning-disabled males were rated significantly lower than a comparison group. The comparison group was also more accurate in assessing its own social status, as learning-disabled subjects tended to overestimate their own popularity. In a second study, with a somewhat larger learning-disabled sample, Bruininks (1978b) obtained essentially the same results: Learning-disabled students were once again rated lower than comparison students, and tended to rate their own status more highly than did other students. Bruininks (1978b) determined that the students with LD could accurately estimate the status of students in the comparison group, thus ruling out response bias (i.e., a tendency to rate everyone more positively) as a factor in the misperception of their own status.

On the other hand, a number of other studies using the peer rating technique have provided results suggesting that not all children with LD have lower-than-normal social status. For example, Perlmutter, Crocker, Cordray, and Garstecki (1983) compared the social status and perceived social status ratings of 55 grade 10 students with LD (identified by the school system) with 107 classmates. Overall, the classmates of these students tended to rate them lower than they rated their normally achieving peers. Classmates also tended to describe students with LD as more aggressive and disruptive. Contrary to the findings of Bruininks (1978a, 1978b), the students with LD were no worse at predicting their social status than were normal students. In addition, Perlmutter et al. (1983) found that about 45% of the students with LD received neutral ratings (not popular, but not disliked); indeed, one subgroup of them (about 20%) was rated quite highly (i.e., within the upper quartile of ratings of normal children) by their peers. In other words, this subgroup of children with LD was as popular as the most popular normal children. Similar results using the nomination method have been reported by Siperstein and Goding (1983).

Some researchers have found that, as a group, children with LD receive social status ratings comparable to those of normal children. For example, Sainato et al. (1983) administered the same rating scale used by Bruininks (1978a, 1978b) to learning-disabled pupils (presumably identified by the school system) and to randomly selected normally achieving classmates. Overall, the range of ratings for the students with LD was comparable to that of the ratings for their classmates. There was also no significant difference in mean ratings for the two groups. Bursuck (1983) has reported comparable results using a nomination technique.

A study by Sabornie and Kauffman (1986) is interesting, not only for the results obtained, but also for a methodological variation that was employed in it. In their investigation, Sabornie and Kauffman selected 46 learning-disabled (identified by an interdisciplinary team within the school system) and matched control secondary school students from coed physical education classes. Peer social status ratings were obtained employing methods similar to those used in other studies, with the exception that "don't know them" responses (which, when provided for, are typically considered neutral responses) were treated separately as a measure of familiarity and did not contribute to social status scores. These investigators found that the social status of learning-disabled students was not significantly different from that of their normal peers. Although the difference in familiarity scores of learning-disabled and normal subjects was not statistically significant, Sabornie and Kauffman (1986) argued that familiarity can impinge on measures of social status, and should be taken into account when assessing social acceptance. When familiarity was taken into consideration in their study, there were no differences in social acceptance between the groups. The authors noted that the outlook for social acceptance of children with LD may not be as bleak as the results of some early studies would seem to suggest.

Finally, Hoyle and Serafica (1988) have reported the results of an investigation using both peer nomination and peer rating methods. In this study, 23 male students with LD (identified by the school's diagnostic team) and matched control subjects were compared on peer nominations and on ratings of "like," "dislike," "neutral," and "unfamiliar" status. A questionnaire examining each child's social network (e.g., number and characteristics of relationships, frequency and type of interactions, etc.) was also administered. Overall, learning-disabled students differed from normal students on the status measures only in terms of the number of peer nominations received. Thus, they were less often named as a best friend, but they were not less liked, more disliked, or more "unfamiliar" than were normally achieving students. Interestingly, learning-disabled subjects less often named as friends those class-mates who expressed liking for them, which suggests that students with LD are less accurate in assessing their own social status, and perhaps have more general problems with social perception. It should be noted, however, that social perception and social status have been found to be only weakly related by Stiliadis and Wiener (in press), and to be unrelated by Bruck and Hebert (1982) and by Martin (1985). With respect to social networks, there was no differ-ence in the size or composition of networks between learning-dis-abled and normal children in the Hoyle and Serafica (1988) study. However, students with LD were less likely to associate with class-mates and to engage in extracurricular activities. The children with LD also spent more time alone or with family members and friends not connected to school, and they also studied more with members of their network (perhaps reflecting a need to work harder at aca-demic subjects).

Teacher Ratings and Interactions

Relatively few studies have involved systematic examinations of the social status of students with LD as perceived by their teachers. Clearly, teachers' perceptions of students with LD may influence their behavior toward these children. That teachers do behave differ-ently toward children with LD has been documented in studies using direct observation. For example, when attempting to initiate interaction with a teacher, children with LD are more likely to be ignored than are normal children (Bryan, 1974a; Bryan & Wheeler, 1972); however, teachers also tend to interact more frequently with learning-disabled students (Dorval, McKinney, & Feagans, 1982), and when they do, they tend to make more negative evaluative statements than they direct to normal children (Bryan, 1974a). Dor-val et al. (1982) found that more than half of teacher-initiated contacts with learning-disabled students involved management of behavior (usually due to inattention or rule breaking), and that these contacts were five times as frequent as similar contacts with normal students. The latter investigators also found that, while students with LD initiated interactions as often as did normal classmates, these contacts were much more likely to be contextually inappropriate (irrelevant and/or disruptive).

Relatively few studies have actually examined teachers' attitudes toward children with LD. In the Perlmutter et al. (1983) study, teachers rated students with LD as less socially competent and as more aggressive and disruptive than their normal classmates (the learning-disabled students' peers rated them similarly; see above). These relations obtained regardless of peer-rated social status. Garrett and Crump (1980) asked teachers to sort students into nine categories (from most to least preferred), and found that learning-disabled students were significantly less preferred than were their normal classmates. Siperstein and Goding (1983) found similar results when they asked teachers to rank students according to overall social performance and classroom behavior. The students with LD were consistently ranked in the lowest third of the class. Using direct observation techniques, Siperstein and Goding (1983) also found that teachers displayed more corrective and nonsupportive/negative behaviors toward students with LD than they did toward normal classmates.

Summary

The available evidence indicates that, as a group, children with LD may have somewhat lower social status than their normally achieving peers. This should not be surprising, as research with non-learning-disabled children has also shown that, in general, academic achievement and social status are positively (but weakly) correlated (Green, Forehand, Beck, & Vosk, 1980). However, it would appear that only some children with LD have truly low social status, and are actively disliked or rejected by peers. On the other hand, some children with LD are quite popular, perhaps because they exhibit attributes that are important to their peers. As they are in most respects, children with LD are heterogeneous with regard to social status. (The importance of considerations relating to the issue of heterogeneity are discussed fully in Chapter 3.) At present, the nature and extent of relations between peer status and other aspects of psychosocial adaptation are poorly understood, as are other predictors and correlates of social status. We arrive at this conclusion despite the assertions of some authors, such as Feigin and Meisgeier (1987), to the contrary. Little is known of teacher perceptions and attitudes toward children with LD; however, the available evidence suggests that further investigation of these potentially important issues is warranted.

Self-Esteem/Self-Concept, and Attributions/Locus of Control

The notion that children with LD are especially likely to be negatively shaped by academic and interpersonal setbacks and failures has been popular for some time. Unfortunately, research in this area has tended to be fragmented, with few investigators detailing the precise theoretical framework in which their research hypotheses have been generated. (See Pickar, 1986, for an example of exceptions to this assertion.) In the interests of clarity, a general model that most investigators in this area appear to espouse is outlined as follows.

Experiences of academic and interpersonal failure result in children with LD developing pathological patterns of attribution and locus of control. For example, such children may come to see their academic and social failure as due to external forces over which they have no control. Alternately, they may see failure as due to their own inadequacies, and their few successes as due to external events (such as luck). Over time, these children come to have reduced self-esteem and poor self-concept (e.g., feelings of inferiority). They may develop patterns of academic and interpersonal behavior that are consistent with "learned helplessness." Poor self-concept, reduced self-esteem, learned helplessness, or other negative effects further interfere with academic and social functioning (possibly by fostering the development of aberrant behaviors), thus exacerbating their psychosocial problems.

There are many variants of this general model, but most research in this area tends to follow, implicitly or explicitly, some form of this line of reasoning. At the same time, we should point out that our literature search did not unearth any investigations that examined all aspects of this model. Most studies have concentrated on rather limited portions of such a model and present the other aspects as "givens," or logical extensions, without providing supporting empirical evidence for such assumptions.

Pathological Self-Esteem/Self-Concept

Obviously, the simplest investigative approach in research following the lines of this model would be to determine whether children with LD do, in fact, evidence reduced self-esteem or pathological self-concepts. In one of the earliest studies addressing this issue, Zimmerman and Allebrand (1965) compared children with roughly normal intellectual abilities who were reading at least 2 years below grade placement to children reading at or above grade level. They found that, overall, the poor readers demonstrated much lower feelings of self-reliance, personal worth, and personal freedom, and greater feelings of anxiety and isolation. The children with reading disability exhibited attitudes toward achievement (as revealed by verbal responses to a projective item) that suggested feelings of discouragement and inadequacy. They also exhibited a tendency to see learning tasks as imposed by authority and without personal benefit.

Empirical results and clinical observations consistent with those of Zimmerman and Allebrand have been reported by a number of investigators. For example, Black (1974) compared matched groups of normal and retarded readers ("retarded reading" was defined as performance at least 6 months below grade level), and found that the retarded readers had lower (more negative) self-concept scores. Black (1974) also found that in both groups, there were significant negative correlations between self-concept and the variables of age, school grade, and measures of reading achievement. Black argued that older students with LD view themselves more negatively than do younger learning-disabled students, and that children tend to judge their personal worth and adequacy on the basis of school performance.

More recently, Margalit and Zak (1984) compared groups of normal children and children with LD (identified by teachers and by brief psychological assessment) on measures of self-concept and anxiety. They found that children with LD showed more "pawning" anxiety (i.e., anxiety regarding events over which they felt they had no control) than did normal children; however, there was no difference between the groups in terms of anxiety over competency issues. Children with LD had lower self-concept scores overall, and they showed a tendency to have greater feelings of self-dissatisfaction.

Winne, Woodlands, and Wong (1982) compared measures of self-concept among groups of normal, gifted, and learning-disabled students who were selected on the basis of tests of vocabulary, reading, and teacher ratings. The self-concept scales covered rather diverse domains, including physical abilities and appearance, intellectual and academic ability, and peer and home relationships. The investigators took some trouble to determine that the inventories were measuring comparable constructs across groups. The results showed that the learning-disabled students exhibited lower evaluations of their own intellectual and academic abilities than did their normal and gifted peers. However, in the other self-concept domains measured, students with LD scored at levels comparable to those of the normal students. Indeed, the learning-disabled students scored significantly higher than did the gifted students in domains related to physical ability and interpersonal relations.

Similar results were found by Chovan and Morrison (1984), who compared groups of learning-disabled, normal, and high-achieving students on six factors of a self-report self-concept inventory. They found that children with LD scored significantly lower (less positively) on two self-concept factors covering behavior and intellectual/school status. However, on factors relating to physical appearance, anxiety, popularity, and happiness, there were no significant differences between the groups.

Academic self-concept and academic expectations of students with LD have also been examined by Hiebert, Wong, and Hunter (1982). In this study, the authors selected learning-disabled and normally achieving students on the basis of identification by school counselors and teachers, who used IQ, achievement test scores, and grade reports. Overall, students with LD, as compared to normal students, reported lower self-concepts relating to academic pursuits and had lower academic expectations. In addition, both the parents and teachers of students with LD had lower academic expectations for these children. The teachers also rated the students with LD as behaving in more socially aberrant ways than normal students behaved.

Unfortunately, many studies, such as that of Chovan and Morrison (1984), provide virtually no information regarding the criteria used to classify children as learning-disabled, and also fail to provide detailed characteristics of the samples used. A demonstration of the desirability of accurately specifying the characteristics of the subjects used is provided by DeFrancesco and Taylor (1985). These investigators noted that previous studies of self-concept in children with LD had ignored two potentially important factors, namely, sex and SES. Both of these dimensions have been shown to have some effect on ratings of self-concept. Thus, these investigators selected two groups of normal and learning-disabled subjects (judged to be so on the basis of standardized testing), and determined both global self-concept (using a self-report scale) and SES (based on parental education, occupation, and residence) of the children. Overall, the investigators found no relationship between sex and self-concept; however, there was a significant correlation between self-concept and SES (specifically, the higher the SES, the higher the self-concept). Although they found that children with LD scored significantly lower on the self-concept measure, SES was found to be a significant covariate accounting for part of the difference between normal and learning-disabled subjects. The authors suggested that differences in socialization practices across social classes may partially mediate differences in self-concept between normally achieving children and children with LD.

Not all investigators have found that children with LD have reduced self-concept/self-esteem, relative to normally achieving peers. For example, Silverman and Zigmond (1983) measured the self-concept of a large sample of middle and high school students classified as learning-disabled on the basis of psychological evaluation. Using a standardized measure of self-concept, they found that their sample of students with LD did not score lower than did the normative sample. They also found no relationship between self-concept and age, IQ, or academic achievement. These findings were confirmed in a second (replication) study contained in the same report. The investigators noted that some individual children within the learning-disabled samples did show rather low self-concept scores. However, the authors concluded that, in general, students with LD do not show reduced self-concept, and that previous findings to the contrary may reflect investigators' prejudices that academic achievement is important in defining self-worth.

Pickar and Tori (1986) have presented findings similar to those of Silverman and Zigmond (1983). In their study, Pickar and Tori examined the issue of self-concept from within an Eriksonian framework: They examined the first six of Erikson's psychosocial stages (trust, autonomy, initiative, industry, identity, and intimacy). They compared normal and learning-disabled secondary school students (diagnosed by means of exclusionary criteria) on a self-concept scale oriented toward the domains of the six Eriksonian psychosocial stages, plus a second commonly used self-concept inventory covering global self-concept and a number of specific domains. Overall, there were few differences between the normal and learning-disabled groups. On the Eriksonian scale, the only difference between groups was in the Industry domain. On the second self-concept scale, students with LD did show lower self-concept scores in the domains of popularity and intellectual/school status; however, the latter was only found in learning-disabled males. The authors concluded that the evidence for lower self-concept in children with LD is equivocal.

Attributions/Locus of Control

Patterns of attributions and locus of control of children with LD have also received some attention from researchers. One contention in such research is that normally achieving students tend to "internalize" success and "externalize" failure (e.g., "I succeed because I am competent; I fail because a task is hard"), whereas children with LD are thought to externalize success and internalize failure (e.g. "I succeed because a task is simple; I fail because I am incompetent"). For example, in an early study of this issue, Hallahan, Gajar, Cohen, and Tarver (1978) found that a group of students with LD demonstrated a significantly greater imputation of degree of external control, relative to a matched group of normal students. These results contrast with those of Hisama (1976), who compared a group of normal children at the third- or fourth-grade level with a group of children identified by teachers, counselors, and principals as having either LD and/or behavior disturbance. This investigator found that there were no differences in locus of control between the normal and special education students. The results of this study suggest that, as a group, children in special education classes (and perhaps children with LD) are no more likely to ascribe failure to internal factors versus external factors than are normal children.

When the special education group in the Hisama (1976) investigation was further subdivided into subgroups with high and low external locus of control, and the performance of these subjects on symbolic transcription tasks was compared, the "low-external" subgroup was found to perform more poorly than did the "high-external" subgroup. Furthermore, when "low-external" children were given negative feedback about their performance on these tests, their performance deteriorated significantly, whereas the performance of the "high-external" subgroup did not change. Thus, it would appear that some special education (and perhaps learning-disabled) children tend to have a more internal locus of control, and that the performance of these children can be adversely affected by negative experiences (Hisama, 1976).

Other researchers have taken a more comprehensive view of attributions in children with LD. For example, Jacobsen, Lowery, and DuCette (1986) noted that some researchers have proposed multidimensional patterns of attributions and behaviors indicative of "learned helplessness" in children with LD as an explanation of academic underachievement. For example, these positions have been maintained in the review papers of Sabatino (1982) and Thomas (1979). These hypothesized patterns of attributions have met with inconsistent, and in some cases contradictory, results on empirical testing. In their own study, Jacobsen et al. (1986) compared patterns of attributions of normal and learning-disabled students under different situations (academic vs. social) and outcomes (success vs. failure). Overall, the results indicated that the children with LD were no more "helpless" than were normal children, as both groups tended to ascribe success to internal factors. However, the children with LD, as compared to the normal children, also tended to invoke the external factors of luck and task ease as explanations for their accomplishments, which might limit feelings of self-worth arising from successful performance. On the other hand, children with LD tended to assume more personal responsibility (i.e., to attribute to themselves lack of effort and ability) in failure situations. Such a pattern of results is inconsistent with a "learned helplessness" model, and the investigators cautioned against attribution remediation efforts based on such an approach (e.g., training children to attribute failure to lack of effort rather than to external, uncontrollable factors).

Other researchers have tried to establish a link between patterns of attribution and self-concept in students with LD. For example, Cooley and Ayres (1988) attempted to relate both self-concept scores and attribution patterns (on internal vs. external and stable vs. unstable dimensions) in groups of normal and learning-disabled students (diagnosed on the basis of intelligence and achievement test scores, and actively receiving special education services). The results showed that the students with LD had lower global self-concept scores than did normal students. However, more detailed analyses indicated that this difference was largely due to differences in self-concept in the academic domain, as had been found in previous studies (see above). Overall, there were no significant differences in attribution patterns between the two groups. However, there was a relationship between attributions and self-concept: Specifically, students with lower self-concept, particularly in the academic domain, tended to attribute success to external factors and failure to inadequate ability (which is a stable internal cause). Cooley and Ayres (1988) argued that such a pattern of attributions and self-concept would produce reduced motivation and effort, leading to feelings of helplessness.

Developmental Considerations

Implicit in the model outlined at the beginning of this section is a developmental dimension: That is, negative academic and interpersonal experiences presumably take time to operate, and may have a cumulative effect on a child (i.e., negative effects become worse with time). This being the case, it is surprising that very few investigations have examined the developmental aspects of this model. One of these few is the study of Chapman and Boersma (1980). These investigators found in a cross-sectional study that achievement expectations, academic self-concept, and locus of control did not differ in learning-disabled students at different grade levels. This would suggest that the negative cognitive–motivational features of children with LD may be stable over time.

In a more recent study, Chapman (1988) followed matched groups of sixth-grade normal and learning-disabled students (selected on the basis of standardized tests and exclusionary criteria) over a 2-year period. At the beginning and end of the study, students were administered an academically oriented locus of control scale, a multidimensional academic self-concept scale, and a multidimensional scale of academic expectations. Overall, the students with LD showed lower self-concept, had lower academic expectations, and demonstrated attribution patterns that suggested a tendency toward learned helplessness (i.e., they were more "externally oriented" with respect to academic achievement). However, these negative cognitive–motivational features of the students with LD did not become worse over time. This finding was particularly interesting as the children in this study were not receiving any special remedial help, and they received significantly lower academic marks over the period of the study than did their normally achieving peers. Thus, despite experiencing continued failure, the children with LD did not show the deterioration in cognitive and motivational features that many investigators might predict.

Thus far, we have examined only studies that have concentrated on the effects of academic experience on attribution, locus of control, and self-esteem/self-concept. Relatively few studies have attempted to demonstrate the effect of experiences outside of the academic domain on these variables. One exception to this generalization is a study conducted by Hall and Richmond (1985). They noted that some previous research had suggested that children with LD have difficulty with nonverbal communication in interpersonal relations. They proposed that such difficulties might be related to reduced self-esteem. Thus, they administered a self-esteem inventory, an interpersonal relations orientation inventory, and a test of perception of nonverbal communication to normal and learning-disabled students (identified as such by the school). They found that children with LD did, in fact, have greater difficulty with nonverbal communication. These students also had lower self-esteem scores overall. However, there was no difference between normal and learning-disabled children with respect to interpersonal orientation; that is, the students with LD reported a comparable need for interpersonal relations (i.e., needs for affection and inclusion). These investigators argued that a normal need for interpersonal relations, coupled with reduced ability to function in those relations (because of problems with nonverbal communication), might be the cause of reduced self-esteem observed in children with LD. These results are consistent with findings reported by Bruininks (1978b).

In a study by Sobol, Earn, Bennett, and Humphries (1983), the attributions and self-concepts of children with LD (selected from clinic referrals on the basis of exclusionary criteria) in social situations were contrasted with those of normal children. Overall, the measure of social self-esteem did not discriminate between normal and learning-disabled subjects. However, these investigators found that the children with LD, as compared to normally achieving children, were more likely to ascribe both positive and negative outcomes in social interactions to luck. The children with LD also had lower expectations of social success than did the normal children. Sobol et al. (1983) argued that these results were consistent with a condition of learned helplessness.

Relationship to Aberrant Behavior

Finally, few investigators have tried to determine whether attributions/locus of control and self-concept are related to aberrant behaviors in children with LD. Some studies, such as that of Pickar and Tori (1986; reviewed above), appear to provide indirect evidence regarding such a relationship. These investigators found that children with LD were no more likely to engage in delinquent behaviors than were normal children, despite finding lower self-concept in some domains in some of the children with LD.

One study that has addressed this issue directly is that of Bender (1987), who examined the in-classroom problem behaviors of normal and learning-disabled students (identified by the school system), and attempted to relate these to measures of self-concept, locus of control, and temperament (task orientation, flexibility, and reactivity). In the learning-disabled group, the relationships between self-concept and locus of control on the one hand, and problem behaviors in the classroom on the other, were generally trivial. Indeed, statistical analyses showed that only 19% of the variance in problem behaviors could be accounted for by the self-concept, locus of control, and temperament measures.

Summary

There is some evidence that some children with LD do demonstrate reduced self-concept with respect to academic (and perhaps intellectual) domains. However, the evidence that children with LD have lower self-concept/self-esteem either globally or in other specific domains is not convincing. There is no evidence that children with LD demonstrate a particular pattern of attributions with respect to success or failure in academic and other settings (see also Bender, 1987). Thus, there is no convincing evidence that in children with LD, reduced self-concept is related to attributions and locus of control. There is no compelling evidence that (1) children with LD demonstrate a pattern of attributions and behaviors consistent with a condition of learned helplessness; (2) self-concept and attribution patterns of LD children are adversely affected by experience of failure; or (3) self-concept and attribution patterns are related to aberrant behavior in children with LD.

Methodological Considerations

Considering the studies reviewed above, we are forced to conclude that research relating to the psychopathology, problems with self-concept/self-esteem, attributions and locus of control, and social status of children with LD has not contributed greatly to our understanding of these children's difficulties. The results of many studies are trivial, contradictory to one another, and not supported in replication attempts. There is little to suggest that the factors identified as "characteristic" of children with LD in these studies are related to one another in any meaningful fashion. In sum, the evidence regarding socioemotional functioning that emerges from the aforementioned research is at best equivocal. A coherent and meaningful pattern of the personality characteristics of children with LD does not emerge from this literature. This may very well be the case because such a pattern does not exist. At this juncture, it is well to point out some of the more obvious methodological inadequacies of this research.

Definition of Learning Disabilities

There has been no consistent formulation of the criteria for LD in these studies. For example, some employed vague or undefined groups, whereas others used the ratings of teachers and other school personnel that remained otherwise unspecified. It is obvious that this lack of clarity and consistency has had a negative impact on the generalizability of such findings. Clear, consensually validatable definitions are vital in this area of investigation.

Measurement of Maladjustment

"Emotional disturbance," "socioemotional adjustment," "behavior disorder," "antisocial behavior," and other constructs of psychosocial functioning have been operationalized as inadequately as "learning disability" in many of these studies, if not more so. It is clear that the use of reliable and valid psychometric instruments would be preferable to the largely subjective judgments of these crucial dependent variables that have characterized much of this research.

Developmental Considerations

Several studies offer support for the notion that the nature of the skill and ability deficits of (some subtypes of) children with LD varies with age (e.g., McKinney, Short, & Feagans, 1985; Morris, Blashfield, & Satz, 1986; Ozols & Rourke, 1988; Rourke, Dietrich, & Young, 1973). Since it would seem reasonable to infer that the socioemotional functioning of (some subtypes of) children with LD would also vary as a function of age (considered as one index of developmental change), the aforementioned inconsistencies in research results may reflect differences in the ages of the subjects employed. To properly investigate this possibility, cross-sectional or longitudinal studies, such as those carried out by Spreen (1988) and colleagues, are necessary.

Heterogeneity

Virtually all of the studies mentioned above have employed a research design that involves comparisons of undifferentiated groups of children with LD to equally undifferentiated groups of normally achieving children. This approach, which aims to identify the particular pattern of socioemotional disturbance characteristic of children with LD, tends to obscure within-group differences. As Applebee (1971) has pointed out, employment of this "comparative-populations" approach can only be justified if one can safely assume that children and adolescents with LD are homogeneous in terms of their abilities and deficits.

Homogeneity of psychosocial functioning, or the lack thereof, has become an increasingly important topic of investigation in recent years. Although some investigators whose work we have reviewed above have noted that not all children with LD behave in a similar manner in the psychosocial domain, discussion of this issue has been largely confined to brief, post hoc descriptions. These descriptions are often couched as explanations for unexpected or contradictory findings, rather than as a proper subject of investigation. However, research into the neuropsychological aspects of LD has suggested strongly that (1) children with LD constitute a markedly heterogeneous population in terms of their skills and abilities, and (2) meaningful subtypes of children with LD can be identified in a reliable fashion with a variety of methods (e.g., Fletcher, 1985; Morris, Blashfield, & Satz, 1981; Rourke & Finlayson, 1978; Rourke & Strang, 1978; Strang & Rourke, 1983).

Apart from our ongoing work at the University of Windsor, which is presented in detail in the next chapter, relatively few systematic attempts to develop a psychosocial typology of children with LD have been reported in the literature. Some fairly recent studies have attempted to identify LD behavioral syndromes by means of R-type factor analysis. Although at first glance this may seem somewhat less appropriate than more direct techniques, such as Q-type factor analysis and cluster analysis, this approach does make some theoretical sense, as both R- and Q-type factor analysis tend to recover the same dimensions when applied to the same data (Lorr, 1983). For example, if R-type factor analysis reveals a "hyperactive" factor in a given data set, Q-type factor analysis on the same data will probably reveal a "hyperactive" subtype (for an example of this point see Fuerst, Fisk, & Rourke, 1989, in which the results of both R- and Q-type factor analyses are reported). This technique has been used with some success in identifying major syndromes of psychopathology in children and adolescents (Achenbach, Conners, Quay, Verhulst, & Howell, 1989).

With respect to learning-disabled populations, this method has been applied to the BPC scores of children with LD. For example, Epstein, Cullinan, and Rosemier (1983) applied principal-components analysis with varimax rotation to the BPC scores of 559 male elementary school students with LD (identified by the school system). The resulting factor structure was similar to that which had been found in previous studies with normal children. Four major factors were identified: Attention Deficit (hyperactive), Anxiety, Conduct Problem, and Social Incompetence.

Epstein, Bursuck, and Cullinan (1985) have also applied principal-components analysis to the BPC scores of 316 older (12 to 18 years) males, 77 older females, and 225 younger (6 to 11 years) females who were identified by their school system as learning-disabled. For all three groups, a Conduct Problem factor was identified as the most salient. An Attention Deficit factor was not found for the older males in the study; instead, items that typically load on this factor merged with the Conduct Problem dimension. The Attention Deficit factor was found in females; however, in older learning-disabled females it tended to have a "flavor" of conduct disorder. In the older males, a Socialized Delinquency factor (e.g., stealing, profanity, fighting, truancy) was found, and a somewhat similar Aggression/Delinquency factor was found in older females. Additional factors of Anxiety–Withdrawal and Inadequacy–Immaturity were found in all three groups. These results suggest that the expression of pathology in children with LD may vary with both age and sex.

Although studies using R-type factor analysis provide interesting information regarding possible dimensions of psychopathology in children with LD, more direct approaches using true statistical classification techniques (e.g., cluster analysis) are required for the development of typologies. A series of studies by McKinney and his colleagues is of considerable interest within this context (see McKinney, 1989, for a detailed summary).

For example, Speece, McKinney, and Appelbaum (1985) were able to classify 63 school-identified children with LD (the average age was approximately 7 years) into seven "behavioral" subtypes by means of one type of cluster analysis. The Classroom Behavior Inventory (CBI; Schaefer, Edgerton, & Aronson, 1977), a rating instrument completed by classroom teachers, was the measure used for clustering. The investigators went to some lengths to examine the internal validity (reliability) and external validity of the subtypes generated. In addition to demonstrating that these learning disability "behavioral" subtypes were different from one another, they showed that the profile patterns generated were quite different from those evident among normally achieving controls. Yet it was also the case that approximately one-third of the children with LD who were classified exhibited profiles on the CBI that were completely normal. Some of the other subtypes generated exhibited profiles that were, at most, within the borderline or very mildly impaired range. It was also the case that subtypes characterized by conduct disorder, withdrawn behavior, and fairly serious, global behavior problems were isolated.

A 3-year longitudinal follow-up of 47 of these youngsters (McKinney & Speece, 1986) yielded evidence of some stability of the subtypes and some change in subtype membership over time. Interestingly, the subtype membership for the children with LD very clearly changed from "normal" to "pathological," or from one "pathological" group to another rather than to the "normal" subtype patterns. Except for the use of a criterion for the determination of LD that is difficult to verify or replicate, and some questionable regrouping of the behavioral subtypes in the longitudinal phases of these studies, these studies are marked by a degree of care and precision that makes for an important contribution to the testing of the assumption of homogeneity.

Social Competence

As has been seen to be the case with the investigations of types of socioemotional disturbance, the experimental hypothesis most often tested in regard to social competence is that of a causal link between it and LD: specifically, that LD lead to deficiencies in social competence. "Social competence" may be conceptualized as a child's ability to satisfy interpersonal needs in ways that are both effective and acceptable to society. The importance of the study of this dimension in children with LD is highlighted by evidence that adult mental health is correlated with childhood social competence (Cowen, Pederson, Babigian, Izzo, & Trost, 1973).

Social competence is difficult to define in operational terms, and researchers interested in determining characteristics of socially competent children (e.g., Nakamura & Finck, 1980) acknowledge the variability of effective social behavior and recognize the importance of situational determinants of such behavior. Nevertheless, the componential analysis of effective social functioning (e.g., Anderson & Messick, 1974; Greenspan, 1981; Gresham & Elliot, 1987; Healey, 1987; Jackson, 1987; Wallander & Hubert, 1987; Weller, Strawser, & Buchanan, 1985) appears to have considerable heuristic value. For example, the large number of skills and abilities identified by a component analysis of social competence can be classified into three groups: (1) perceptual skills, such as those needed for the perception of facial expressions; (2) cognitive abilities, such as those required to discern cause-and-effect relations in social events; and (3) motor and language skills, by which children manifest their social behavior. Competent social behavior can be seen as a result of a complex interaction and coordination of these and related variables. It is also widely held that attitudinal characteristics, such as differentiated self-concept and consolidation of identity, a concept of oneself as an initiating and controlling agent, and a realistic appraisal of oneself, accompanied by feelings of personal worth, are crucial factors in the development of social competence.

As outlined in detail above, literature in the LD area reveals frequent claims that such children experience problems in their social relationships, and that their socioemotional difficulties persist into adolescence and adulthood (e.g., Bryan, Donohue, & Pearl, 1981; Kronick, 1980; Siegel, 1974). Variables that have been utilized to investigate the validity of such claims include parent observations (Owen, Adams, Forrest, Stolz, & Fisher, 1971), teacher ratings (Bryan & McGrady, 1972; Keogh, Tchir, & Windeguth-Behn, 1974; Margalit, 1989), peer ratings (Bryan, 1974b), classroom observations of the interactions of students with LD (Bryan, 1974a; Bryan & Wheeler, 1972), and behavior checklists (McConaughy & Ritter,

1986). The results of these studies have demonstrated that in comparison to their normally achieving peers, youngsters with LD tend to be judged in more negative and rejecting terms by parents, teachers, and classmates, and/or that they are perceived as much less competent in social adaptation. Some studies have also shown that some children with LD may be relatively deficient in perceiving their own social status (Bruininks, 1978b).

Explanations for these deficiencies have usually focused on a single perceptual, cognitive, or behavioral skill that is said to be lacking in children with LD. For example, various investigators have searched for the following: a schematic judgment deficit, or an inability to realize the organization of an interactional situation (Kronick, 1980); deficits in role-taking skills (Bruck & Hebert, 1982); a linguistic deficit that results in poor interpersonal communication skills and problems in understanding the rules that govern socially appropriate speech (Bryan, 1982); deficits in emitted nonverbal signals (Raskind, Drew, & Regan, 1983); abnormal interpersonal goals and strategies (Carlson, 1987); and deficits in the ability to draw appropriate inferences from nonverbal stimuli (Gerber & Zinkgraf, 1982). Other studies have investigated the ability of children with LD to perceive and interpret accurately the affective states of others. Ability to label emotions expressed through nonverbal means (Axelrod, 1982; Wiig & Harris, 1974), to select appropriate facial expressions for material presented in stories (Bachara, 1976), and to describe emotional scenarios from videotaped displays of emotion (Bryan, 1977; Pearl & Cosden, 1982; Stone & LaGreca, 1984; Weiss, 1984) have been examined, with inconsistent results.

There would appear to be at least two major reasons why the results of these studies do not contribute a great deal to the testing of Hypothesis 2, as follows (elements of each of these are alluded to by LaGreca, 1981, 1987):

1. *Lack of a conceptual model.* There is an obvious absence in these studies of a conceptual model to elucidate the skills involved in social competence that are deficient in children with LD (see Goldman & Hardin, 1982, for an example of this problem). (A notable exception to this is the formulation of Wiener, 1980.) For example, at the very minimum, a componential analysis of social competence should sensitize the researcher to the possibility that, whereas some subtypes of children with LD may experience social

competence problems because they lack certain perceptual, cognitive, or behavioral skills, others may manifest such problems as a more direct result of attitudinal/motivational difficulties. It should also be clear that different patterns of perceptual, cognitive, and behavioral skills and abilities may encourage different types or degrees of socially incompetent behavior.

2. *Definitional problems and subtypes.* Related to the first point is the use of inconsistent and/or unclear definitions of LD in these studies, and an almost total lack of sensitivity to the notion that there may be subtypes of children with LD who may find various types of social competence more or less difficult to achieve. Notable exceptions to the latter problem are the work of Loveland, Fletcher, and Bailey (1990), McConaughty and Ritter (1986), and, to a lesser extent, Silver and Young (1985).

An example of research (Ozols & Rourke, 1985) that has attempted to grapple with some of these difficulties is presented below. First, however, it is necessary to place this particular piece of research within the context of a general approach to the neuropsychological investigation of central processing abilities and deficits in learning-disabled and frankly brain-damaged youngsters that gave rise to this type of investigation.

It is unfortunate that the utilization of a neuropsychological framework for this purpose has so often been misinterpreted as reflecting an emphasis on static, intractable (and therefore limited) notions of the effects of brain impairment on behavior. Indeed, although specific statements to the contrary have been made on many occasions (e.g., Rourke, 1975, 1978b), many otherwise competent researchers and clinicians persist in the notion that such an approach assumes that brain damage, disorder, or dysfunction lies at the basis of LD. Nothing could be further from the truth, since the aim of much work in this area (see reviews by Benton, 1975, and Rourke, 1978a) has been to demonstrate whether and to what extent such might be the case.

Be that as it may, the emphasis of a neuropsychological approach is to attempt to integrate dimensions of social and emotional development on the one hand with relevant central processing features on the other, in order to fashion a useful model by which to study crucial aspects of individual human development, including LD. That models and explanatory concepts developed with this aim in mind (e.g., Rourke, 1976, 1982, 1983, 1987) contain explanations that are thought to apply both to some types of frankly brain-damaged and learning-disabled children *and* to some aspects of normal human development should come as no surprise, since maximum generalizability is one goal of any scientific model or theory. Specifically, with respect to the child with LD, the most relevant aspects of these concepts and models are those that have to do with proposed linkages between patterns of central processing abilities and deficits that may predispose a youngster to predictably different patterns of social as well as academic LD. In addition, these models are designed to encompass developmental change and outcome in patterns of learning and behavioral responsivity.

For example, since 1971 at the University of Windsor, we have been investigating two subtypes of children with LD; these subtypes were the focus of investigation in the Ozols and Rourke (1985) study. Children in one group (referred to as Group R-S) are those who exhibit many relatively poor psycholinguistic skills in conjunction with very well-developed abilities in visual–spatial–organizational, tactile–perceptual, psychomotor, and nonverbal problem-solving skills. They exhibit very poor reading and spelling skills, and significantly better (though still impaired) mechanical arithmetic competence. The other group (Group A) exhibits outstanding problems in visual–spatial–organizational, tactile–perceptual, psychomotor, and nonverbal problem-solving skills, within a context of clear strengths in some psycholinguistic skills such as rote verbal learning, regular phoneme–grapheme matching, amount of verbal output, and verbal classification. Group A children experience their major academic learning difficulties in mechanical arithmetic, while exhibiting advanced levels of word recognition and spelling. Both of these subtypes of children with LD—especially the second (Group A) subtype, characterized as having "nonverbal learning disabilities"—have been the subject of much scrutiny in our laboratory (for reviews, see Rourke, 1975, 1978b, 1982, 1987, 1989; Rourke & Strang, 1983; Strang & Rourke, 1985a, 1985b). The results of one of the studies in this series (Ozols & Rourke, 1985) are of particular relevance with respect to the investigation of social competence; the relevant aspects of this investigation may be summarized as follows.

The performances of two groups of children with LD—one exhibiting a pattern of relatively poor auditory-perceptual and language-related skills within a context of well-developed visual–spatial–organizational skills (similar to Group R-S), and the second exhibiting the opposite pattern of abilities and deficits (similar to Group A)—were compared on four exploratory measures of social judgment and responsiveness. As predicted on the basis of the Rourke (1982) model, one result of this study revealed that children in the language disorder group performed more effectively than did those in the visual–spatial disorder group on tasks requiring nonverbal responses; in contrast, tasks requiring verbal responses yielded exactly the opposite results. These results suggest that social awareness and responsiveness vary markedly for these two subtypes of children with LD, probably as a result of an interaction between their particular patterns of central processing abilities and deficits and the specific task demands of the four measures employed.

A recent study by Loveland et al. (1990) has replicated and extended these findings. In this investigation, three groups of children were employed: nondisabled, Group R-S, and Group A. They were compared on tasks requiring verbal (description) and nonverbal (enactment) comprehension and production of verbally and nonverbally presented stories that included significant affective and motivational components. In general, Group R-S children encountered greatest difficulty when asked to describe the verbally presented stories, whereas Group A children had the greatest difficulty when asked to enact the nonverbally presented stories. When stories were presented nonverbally, Group A children showed a greater tendency to reverse the roles of characters and to omit or misinterpret events. Although both Group R-S and Group A children had more difficulty interpreting motivation and affect in the stories than nondisabled children did, there was a strong tendency for Group A children to make the greatest number of motivational and affective misinterpretations.

The results of the Ozols and Rourke (1985) and Loveland et al. (1990) studies should be viewed within the context of a study by Ackerman and Howes (1986). This study demonstrated that although social competence deficits often occur in many children with LD, it is the case that some children with LD do not exhibit such deficits and are seen as popular with their peers and active in after-school interests. These findings, taken together, would suggest that a study designed along the lines of the Porter and Rourke (1985;

see Chapter 3) investigation may reveal an analogous set of "social competence" subtypes (i.e., some children are "normal" and others "disturbed" in terms of social competence). (The studies by Speece et al., 1985, and McKinney & Speece, 1986, contain some data that could be used to address this question directly.) It is clear that, as in the case of the investigation of emotional disturbance in youngsters with LD, the examination of their social competence should eschew the homogeneous, contrasting-groups methodology that has heretofore characterized all but a few studies in the field, in favor of one that does justice to the heterogeneity of subtypes evident in the learning-disabled population.

Furthermore, it would appear to be the case that efforts to relate patterns of abilities and deficits on the one hand and components of social competence on the other may generate much more interesting data and conclusions than do approaches that simply search for correlates of LD (considered as a univocal phenomenon) and either emotional disturbance or problems in social competence. The studies reviewed in connection with the examination of Hypothesis 3 constitute another step beyond the latter type of simplistic contrasting-groups/unitary-deficit methodologies.

3

The Windsor
Taxonomic Research

Before turning our attention to the most recent formulations of the
psychosocial functioning of children with learning disabilities
(LD), the so-called Hypothesis 3 approaches, we examine in detail
one issue raised in the preceding chapter: heterogeneity. At this
point in our review, it should be apparent that much of the research
in this area has produced confusing and contradictory results. For
some time we have suspected that this is due in large part to the use
of variants of the simple contrasting-groups design, in which an
undifferentiated group of children with LD is compared to an
equally undifferentiated group of normally achieving children. The
assumption underlying this design is that all children with LD may
be susceptible to developing a particular pattern of psychosocial
dysfunction, and that within-group differences are of little concern.
This method can only be justified if the assumption that children
with LD comprise a homogeneous group with respect to psychosocial functioning is valid.

In our laboratory, we have undertaken a research program with
the immediate aim of more precisely describing the psychosocial
functioning of children with LD. This chapter provides an overview
of a series of five studies in which we and our colleagues have
systematically explored patterns of personality and psychosocial
functioning in children with LD. In these studies, we have applied
multivariate statistical subtyping methods, such as Q-type factor
analysis and some of the many variants of cluster analysis, to se-

lected scales of the Personality Inventory for Children (PIC; Wirt, Lachar, Klinedinst, & Seat, 1977, 1984), in an attempt to derive both reliable and valid psychosocial subtypes of children with LD. These studies are the initial steps in a comprehensive research program aimed at the development of a psychosocial typology of children with LD; for want of a better term, we refer to them as the "Windsor Taxonomic Research." Note that in this chapter we concentrate on describing the subtyping techniques that we have used, and the characteristics of the typology that has emerged from this research. Other aspects of these studies are more germane to issues raised in the next chapter (Hypothesis 3 approaches) and are presented there within that context.

STUDY 1

In the first study of this series, Porter and Rourke (1985) investigated whether the assumption of psychosocial homogeneity can be justified on an empirical basis by application of a multivariate statistical subtyping technique (Q-type factor analysis) to the PIC scores of 100 children with LD. On the basis of the resulting factor pattern, 77 children were assigned to one of four subtypes; the subtypes were then examined in terms of the mean PIC profiles exhibited by the subjects within them.

The first and largest subtype (the "Normal" subtype, including about half of the subjects) showed no elevations on PIC scales reflecting psychosocial disturbance, and had an essentially well-adjusted profile. The parents of these children were most concerned with the cognitive development and academic functioning of their children. The second subtype (the "Internalized Psychopathology" subtype, including about one-quarter of the subjects) had a mean PIC profile that was strongly suggestive of seriously disturbed socioemotional functioning of an internalized type (e.g., symptoms suggestive of depression, withdrawal, and anxiety). The third subtype (the "Externalized Psychopathology" subtype, with about 15% of the subjects) had a mean PIC profile that was suggestive of externalized, hyperkinetic behavioral disturbance. The fourth and smallest group derived (the "Somatic Concern" subtype, with about 10% of subjects) showed relatively normal psychosocial adjustment overall, but evidenced a variety of somatic complaints. As the four subtypes derived through Q-type factor analysis exhibited clearly different patterns of psychosocial functioning, Porter and Rourke (1985) concluded that the personality characteristics of children with LD are heterogeneous, and that there is no unique LD personality type.

STUDY 2

Statistical subtyping techniques, such as Q-type factor analysis and cluster analysis, will always produce some grouping of observations, even if purely random data are input to the techniques. Thus, in the next study in this series, we (Fuerst, Fisk, & Rourke, 1989) concentrated on establishing the reliability (also known as "replicability" or "internal validity") of the Porter and Rourke (1985) subtypes, using a new sample of children and a variety of statistical subtyping techniques. The scores of 132 children with LD, between the ages of 6 and 12 years, on nine selected PIC scales were investigated using Q-type factor analysis, four hierarchical–agglomerative clustering techniques, and one iterative partitioning clustering technique. The results revealed excellent correspondence between the subtypes derived by all grouping methods, in terms of both misclassifications and mean PIC profile similarity of the subtypes across techniques.

   Three subtypes were found in the study. The mean PIC profile of one subtype indicated normal psychosocial adjustment. This group was almost identical to the Normal children reported by Porter and Rourke (1985) in terms of both general PIC profile shape and elevation, and relative size. The second subtype exhibited evidence of significant internalized psychopathology, and was very similar to the corresponding subtype of children found in the Porter and Rourke (1985) study. There were only trivial discrepancies in mean profiles between the Internalized Psychopathology subtypes that were generated in the two studies; these were greatly overshadowed by overall similarity of shape and general elevation. The relative sizes of the two groups were also comparable. The third subtype had a mean PIC profile suggestive of externalized, hyperkinetic psychopathology, and was very similar to the corresponding

Porter and Rourke (1985) subtype. The profile of this group also bore a striking resemblance to one reported by Breen and Barkley (1983) in a study of 26 children diagnosed as hyperactive or as having Attention Deficit Disorder with Hyperactivity. Indeed, the two profiles were highly correlated ($r = .89$), confirming substantial similarity of profile shape. The fourth subtype of Porter and Rourke (1985), Somatic Concern, was not found in this study.

The results of the Porter and Rourke (1985) and Fuerst et al. (1989) studies led to three important conclusions. First, children with LD are heterogeneous in terms of psychosocial functioning; that is, there is no unique LD personality type. Second, statistical subtyping techniques can produce reliable and interpretable subgroups of children that are replicable across samples. Third, LD children seem to fall into three broad psychosocial subtypes— namely, Normal, Internalized Psychopathology, and Externalized Psychopathology. About half of the children studied demonstrated the first pattern of psychosocial functioning, with the remainder being divided between the latter two patterns.

STUDY 3

Although these three general patterns of psychosocial functioning are consistent with patterns of PIC profiles seen in clinical practice, experience would suggest that a greater diversity of psychosocial functioning is in fact presented by children with LD. In the next study (Fuerst, Fisk, & Rourke, 1990), more sophisticated clustering techniques and a somewhat wider range of PIC scales were used to develop a more fine-grained typology of psychosocial functioning. The same 132 children who took part in the Fuerst et al. (1989) investigation were used in this study.

In this investigation, six, rather than three, subtypes were identified within the sample. These could be readily replicated with a variety of clustering methods. One subtype (Normal) exhibited a mean PIC profile that suggested good psychosocial functioning, with elevations only on scales related to academic and intellectual functioning, and was very strongly related to the Fuerst et al. (1989) Normal group. A second subtype was also relatively well adapted, with some indications of mild hyperactive or acting-out forms of behavior ("Mild Hyperactive"). A third subtype was characterized chiefly by elevation of the PIC Somatic Concern scale. This subtype was not related to any of the three found in the Fuerst et al. (1989) study, but was very similar to the Somatic Concern group found by Porter and Rourke (1985). Two of the subtypes were related to the Internalized Psychopathology group found in Fuerst et al. (1989): One subtype showed evidence of mild anxiety and depression (labeled "Mild Anxiety"), while the other showed evidence of severe internalized psychopathology. Finally, an Externalized Psychopathology or hyperactive subtype, very similar to that in the Fuerst et al. (1989) study, was also found. (The results of this study that relate to Wechsler Intelligence Scale for Children [WISC] Verbal–Performance IQ discrepancies are discussed in Chapter 4, which deals with Hypothesis 3.)

STUDY 4

In the fourth study of this series, we (Fuerst & Rourke, 1991a) attempted to replicate the subtypes found in Fuerst et al. (1990) in a large and diverse sample of children. In this investigation, the subjects were 500 children between the ages of 6 and 12 years, with normal psychometric intelligence and (to ensure an adequate sample of psychopathology) at least one PIC clinical scale score greater than 70 *T*. The subjects were clustered by the *k*-means method, using the same PIC scales that were employed in Fuerst et al. (1990). The result was six subtypes, five of which were extremely similar to the subtypes found in the latter study (viz., Normal, Somatic Concern, Mild Anxiety, Internalized Psychopathology, and Externalized Psychopathology). In this study, a Mild Hyperactive group was not found; however, a sixth subtype (labeled "Conduct Disorder") did have a mean PIC profile suggestive of conduct disorder.

STUDY 5

In the final study of this series, we (Fuerst & Rourke, 1991b) attempted to explore the relations between age and patterns of psychosocial functioning. To this end, a sample of 728 children with LD between the ages of 7 and 13 years was constructed. All children met a commonly used set of criteria for LD, which included normal intelligence, evidence of underachievement on a standardized test of academic skills, and no evidence of primary psychopathology (as judged by the clinician having principal responsibility for the case). For some analyses, children were subdivided into three age levels: "young" (7-8 years old; 201 subjects), "middle" (9-10 years; 258 subjects), and "old" (11-13 years; 269 subjects).

As in Studies 1 through 4, psychosocial functioning was defined by scores on the PIC. Two methods were used for derivation of psychosocial subtypes. The first method employed *k*-means cluster analysis, applied separately to each of the young, middle, and old samples, using a dissimilarity measure calculated on 10 PIC scales transformed in a manner that emphasizes profile shape over the elements of elevation and dispersion. The resulting *k*-means partitions were validated by replication, using a variety of hierarchical-agglomerative clustering techniques.

The subtypes derived by cluster analysis (referred to as "cluster-analysis-derived" [CAD] subtypes) at each of the three age levels were very similar, and were strongly related to clusters found in Studies 1-4. At all three age levels, Normal, Internalized Psychopathology, and Externalized Psychopathology subtypes were found. Although there were minor differences between corresponding subtypes across age levels, they were all clearly recognizable as instances of their respective types, which suggests that the major *patterns* of psychosocial functioning are consistent across ages 7 through 13. In addition, the finding that the Internalized Psychopathology and Externalized Psychopathology CAD subtypes were very similar across the young, middle, and old samples also suggests that with increased age there is no change in the *level* of pathology evidenced in frankly maladjusted subtypes. There was no evidence of greater maladjustment in these two clearly pathological subtypes at higher age levels.

There was no evidence of greater diversity of subtypes at higher age levels. Whereas more subtypes were found in the middle sample (six) than in the young sample (four), only four subtypes could be reliably derived from the old sample. The discrepancy in the number of subtypes across age levels (four vs. six) was trivial. These results also suggest that patterns of psychosocial functioning, as measured by the PIC, are quite uniform from 7 to 13 years of age in children with LD.

A second method of classification used in Study 5 involved assigning subjects to the subtypes of a prototypical typology derived in previous research, on the basis of similarity of PIC profile shape. As outlined above, previous research in our laboratory (Studies 1 through 4) has produced a typology of seven psychosocial subtypes (viz., Normal, Somatic Concern, Mild Anxiety, Mild Hyperactive, Conduct Disorder, Internalized Psychopathology, and Externalized Psychopathology) based on PIC scores. Calculating the mean PIC scores on all 16 scales for the seven previously derived subtypes resulted in the creation of "prototypical" PIC profiles for those subtypes. Next, correlations between each subject's PIC profile and the seven prototypical PIC profiles were calculated, and subjects were assigned ("matched") to the subtypes to which their PIC profiles correlated most strongly.

When the subtypes derived from profile matching (referred to as "profile-matching-derived" [PMD] subtypes) were further broken down at the young, middle, and old age levels, there were no substantial differences between the resulting mean PIC profiles, in terms of either profile shape or elevation, within each subtype. There was an extremely slight tendency for old subjects to be found more frequently in the Conduct Disorder and Internalized Psychopathology subtypes, although the validity of this finding was questionable.

SUMMARY OF STUDIES 1 THROUGH 5

Internal Validity (Reliability) of the Typology

The results of the five studies reviewed above are summarized schematically in Figure 3.1. Each box on the chart represents a subtype derived from the source noted in the leftmost column of the figure. Within each box is a descriptive label that characterizes the mean PIC profile of the subtype, and, in the lower right corner, the relative size of the subtype is expressed as a percentage of the subjects classified within the study. Correlations between corresponding subtypes across studies appear on the connecting lines. Note that, although some of the subtypes are arranged hierarchically, this order is based on the *temporal* course of our research and is not meant to imply that such a hierarchical division does in fact exist. Whether certain broad categories of psychosocial functioning can be usefully and accurately divided into subcategories, as implied by the figure, can only be determined by further research.

The first four rows of the figure present the subtypes found in Studies 1 through 4: Porter and Rourke (1985), Fuerst et al. (1989), Fuerst et al. (1990), and Fuerst and Rourke (1991a). The fifth row ("Overall Studies 1–4") summarizes the typology that emerged across those four studies. In this case, the relative size values represent the average percentages of subjects assigned to subtypes across the four studies. The final four rows of the figure present the results from Study 5 (Fuerst & Rourke, 1991b). The results of that study are broken down into young CAD subtypes, middle CAD subtypes, old CAD subtypes, and PMD subtypes derived from the entire sample. In this portion of the figure, the correlations on connecting lines represent the correlation between the mean PIC profile of the subtype and the corresponding prototype developed from Studies 1 through 4.

Ideally, subtyping methods of any type should produce reliable, homogeneous groups that can be replicated across different samples and classification techniques (Everitt, 1980). This issue is of particular concern when multivariate subtyping techniques are applied in an exploratory fashion to data with relatively unknown statistical properties. Multivariate subtyping techniques, such as cluster analysis and Q-type factor analysis, will always produce some grouping of cases, even if purely random data are used in the procedures; moreover, different statistical subtyping techniques can (and often do) produce disparate solutions when applied to the same data. Replicability of solutions across different samples from the same population, and across different subtyping techniques, is a crucial step in determining the validity of the subtypes so derived (Fletcher, 1985). When the results of Studies 1 through 5 are considered, it is apparent that four of the subtypes are readily replicable with different samples, statistical techniques, and sets of PIC scales.

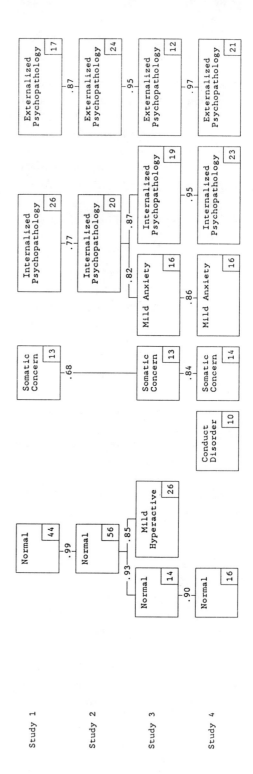

56

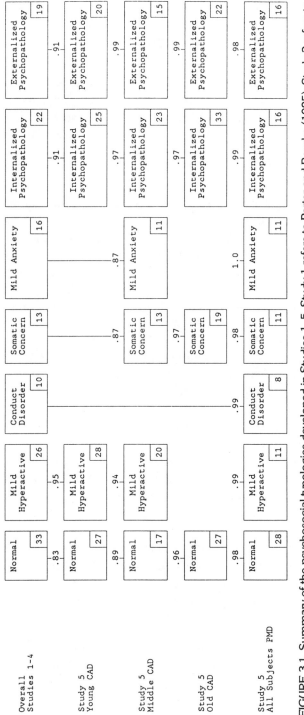

FIGURE 3.1. Summary of the psychosocial typologies developed in Studies 1–5. Study 1 refers to Porter and Rourke (1985); Study 2 refers to Fuerst, Fisk, and Rourke (1989); Study 3 refers to Fuerst, Fisk, and Rourke (1990); Study 4 refers to Fuerst and Rourke (1991a); and Study 5 refers to Fuerst and Rourke (1991b). See text for further explanation.

Perhaps the most reliable subtype that has been found is the Externalized Psychopathology or hyperactive group. This subtype was found in all five studies (counting the three age levels used in Fuerst & Rourke, 1991b, there are six samples in total). Furthermore, in all studies the mean PIC profiles of instances of this subtype have been very consistent. The relative size (or the percentage of assigned subjects found in the subtype; summarized in Figure 3.1) of the Externalized Psychopathology subtype has also been very stable across studies (about 15%–25%).

The second most consistent subtype has been the Internalized Psychopathology cluster. Like the Externalized Psychopathology subtype, this group has been found in all studies to date (six samples). The mean PIC profiles of the instances of this subtype have been very consistent across studies, and there have only been trivial deviations in the percentage of subjects assigned to it (overall, about 20%–25%).

The third most consistent subtype has been the Normal group. This subtype has also been in evidence in all previous investigations (six samples). In all studies the instances of the Normal subtype have been quite similar across samples, with the exception that in Study 5 (Fuerst & Rourke, 1991b), the young CAD Normal subtype evidenced some minor peaks on the PIC Somatic Concern and Delinquency scales. With respect to the percentage of subjects assigned to the subtype, there has been some variance in the relative size of this subtype from study to study. Across Studies 1 through 4, on average about 33% of subjects have been assigned to this subtype, and similar values were found for the young and old CAD subtypes in Study 5. However, the relative sizes of the Study 3 (Fuerst et al., 1990), Study 4 (Fuerst & Rourke, 1991a), and Study 5 (Fuerst & Rourke, 1991b) middle CAD instances of the subtype were only about half as large. It is important to note that in these three cases the typologies included a relatively large number of subtypes (six, vs. three or four). This pattern suggests that, when subtypes are formed using cluster analysis (with a greater number of subtypes formed and finer discriminations made between patterns of psychosocial functioning), subjects who might be classified as Normal in relatively coarse typologies do show some differences, perhaps contributing (to an as yet unknown extent) to the Mild Hyperactive, Conduct Disorder, or Mild Anxiety groups. In any event, these latter three subtypes clearly demonstrate mild degrees of psychosocial disturbance, and they are much more similar to the Normal subtype than they are to the severely disturbed Internalized and Externalized Psychopathology subtypes.

The fourth most reliable subtype found to date is Somatic Concern. Although this subtype was not found in Study 2 (Fuerst et al., 1989) or in the young CAD typology of Study 5 (Fuerst & Rourke, 1991b), it has been found in five different samples of children with LD. Across all studies, the mean PIC profile of instances of this subtype has been very consistent. In terms of relative size, the percentage of subjects assigned to the Somatic Concern subtype has been roughly equivalent across studies (about 14%).

Some evidence suggests (but does not establish) that two of the remaining seven subtypes, Mild Hyperactive and Mild Anxiety, have some internal validity (reliability). The Mild Hyperactive subtype was first derived in Study 3 (Fuerst et al., 1990; note that this single instance of the subtype constitutes the prototype). Although it was not replicated in Study 4 (Fuerst & Rourke, 1991a), a Mild Hyperactive subtype did appear in the young and middle CAD typologies of Study 5 (Fuerst & Rourke, 1991b). The mean PIC profiles of these two instances of the subtype were very similar to the prototypical Mild Hyperactive PIC profile, as were the percentages of assigned subjects (26%, 28%, and 20% for the Study 3 sample and the Study 5 young and middle samples, respectively).

The Mild Anxiety subtype has been found in three samples to date (Fuerst et al., 1990; Fuerst & Rourke, 1991a; Fuerst & Rourke, 1991b, middle sample). The mean PIC profiles of these instances of the subtype have been very similar across studies. In addition, the percentage of assigned subjects found in the subtype has been roughly consistent across these samples (overall, about 15%).

The least reliable subtype is Conduct Disorder. This group has been derived using cluster analysis in only one study to date, Study 4 (Fuerst & Rourke, 1991a). A Conduct Disorder subtype very similar to that found in Study 4 was derived using profile matching in Study 5 (Fuerst & Rourke, 1991b). The relative size of the PMD Conduct Disorder subtype (8%) was comparable to that found in Study 4 (10%). However, until this subtype is replicated in a new sample of children, its reliability will remain suspect.

Description of the Typology

Note that the correlation coefficients in Figure 3.1 (calculated between the mean PIC profiles of the subtypes) were used to match corresponding subtypes across the five studies. Overall, across Studies 1 through 5, seven distinct subtypes (viz., Normal, Mild Hyperactive, Mild Anxiety, Somatic Concern, Conduct Disorder, Internalized Psychopathology, and Externalized Psychopathology) have been identified. Averaging the PIC scores of corresponding subtypes across studies (e.g., PIC scores of all of the Normal subtypes) makes it possible to obtain "prototypical" mean PIC profiles for the seven subtypes. Prototypical profiles are presented in Figures 3.2 to 3.8. (Note that these figures were derived from the subtypes generated in Studies 1–4. The data reported in Study 5 are so new that the prototypes in Figures 3.2 through 3.8 could not be updated in time for this writing. Visual inspection of the mean PIC profiles from Study 5, and the correlation coefficients between the Study 5 subtypes and the prototypes derived from Studies 1–4 [reported in Figure 3.1], suggest strongly that addition of the Study 5 data will not significantly alter the profiles found in Figures 3.2 through 3.8.)

Of course, presentation of PIC profiles without interpretation does not describe behavior, as the scale labels are, in some respects, arbitrary. For example, elevation of the Psychosis scale above 70 T does not mark a child as psychotic. Similarly, the labels given to the subtypes, such as Normal or Mild Hyperactive, have been used more as descriptions of the pattern of scores on the mean PIC profiles than as descriptions of behavior. For example, the PIC profile of the Normal subtype is in fact abnormal, with clinically meaningful elevations on some PIC scales. However, elevations on the Academic Achievement, Intellectual Screening, and Development scales in the context of an otherwise roughly flat profile are unremarkable, or "normal" with respect to psychosocial disturbance, in samples of children with LD.

In this section, the subtypes are discussed in terms of psychosocial adaptation, or general patterns of behavioral function–dysfunction that would be expected on the basis of our current understanding of the PIC. Note that these characterizations are actually *expectations* or predictions that, in the process of establishing the external validity of the typology, must be tested in future research.

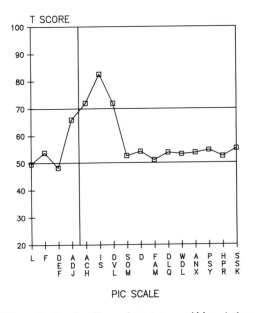

FIGURE 3.2. PIC profile for the Normal prototype. Abbreviations for Figures 3.2–3.8 are as follows: L, Lie; DEF, Defensiveness; ADJ, Adjustment; ACH, Achievement; IS, Intellectual Screening; DVL, Development; SOM, Somatic Concern; D, Depression; FAM, Family Relations; DLQ, Delinquency; WDL, Withdrawal; ANX, Anxiety; PSY, Psychosis; HPR, Hyperactivity; and SSK, Social Skills.

Note also that for the sake of clarity in the following descriptions, minor variations in the profiles of subtypes with the same labels (e.g., Somatic Concern), but derived from different studies and samples and using different methods (cluster analysis vs. Q-type factor analysis vs. profile matching), have been ignored, and the most salient features have been emphasized.

Two of the subtypes have mean PIC profiles that suggest relatively good psychosocial functioning. The profile of the Normal subtype (Figure 3.2) shows mean elevations above 70 *T* on the Achievement, Intellectual Screening, and Development scales (the so-called "cognitive triad"—a pattern found, to a greater or lesser extent, in all subtypes), and a very flat profile on all other clinical scales. The caretakers of these children are most concerned with

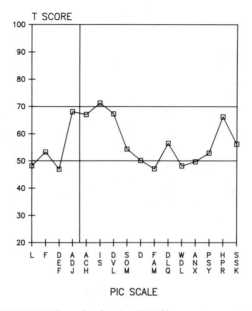

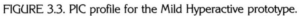

FIGURE 3.3. PIC profile for the Mild Hyperactive prototype.

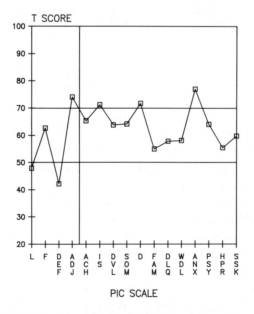

FIGURE 3.4. PIC profile for the Mild Anxiety prototype.

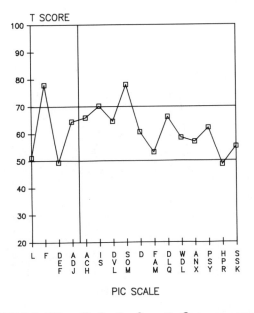

FIGURE 3.5. PIC profile for the Somatic Concern prototype.

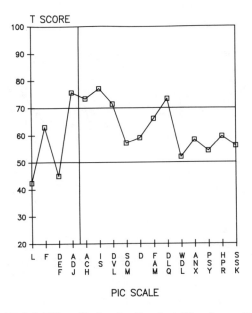

FIGURE 3.6. PIC profile for the Conduct Disorder prototype.

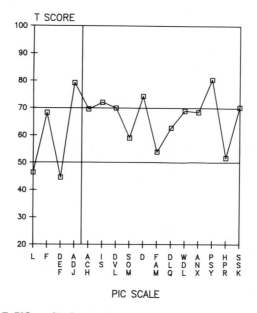

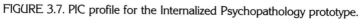

FIGURE 3.7. PIC profile for the Internalized Psychopathology prototype.

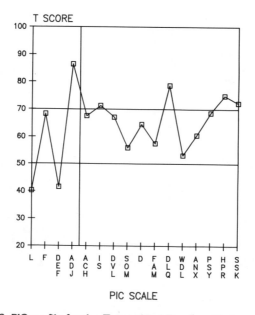

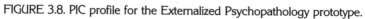

FIGURE 3.8. PIC profile for the Externalized Psychopathology prototype.

cognitive development and academic performance. The mean PIC profile of the Somatic Concern subtype (Figure 3.5) is similar to that of the Normal subtype, but it is marked by elevation of the Somatic Concern scale. The caretakers of these children are likely to express distress about the children's physical well-being and health. Physical complaints may span a wide range of difficulties, including visual problems, dizziness, headaches, syncope, fatigue, and gastrointestinal dysfunction. However, it should be noted that, as with other psychosocial measures tapping somatic domains, it is not possible to determine the degree to which such complaints may be functional rather than "organic" in nature, on the basis of the PIC profile alone. Elevation on this scale may be more indicative of a need for medical assessment (e.g., for otitis media) and intervention than of psychosocial dysfunction.

Two of the subtypes evidence modest degrees of psychosocial dysfunction. Children in the Mild Hyperactive subtype (Figure 3.3) show a relatively unremarkable PIC profile that is distinguished by a single significant elevation above 70 T on the Intellectual Screening scale, and a somewhat higher than usual mean score on the Hyperactivity scale. This suggests fairly good psychosocial adaptation in most domains, as in the Normal subtype, with the possibility of rather mild acting-out behaviors. The profile of the Mild Anxiety subtype (Figure 3.4) also suggests mild psychosocial disturbance, with notable (but relatively modest) peaks on the Intellectual Screening, Depression, and Anxiety scales. Overall, this profile suggests symptoms of mild anxiety and depression, and is somewhat reminiscent of the PIC profile of the Internalized Psychopathology subtype.

In some respects, the PIC profile of the Conduct Disorder subtype (Figure 3.6) also suggests relatively mild psychosocial dysfunction, with a single peak on the Delinquency scale. However, the behaviors that may be demonstrated by such children are likely to be more problematic for caretakers and peers than are those demonstrated by children in the Mild Hyperactive or Mild Anxiety subtypes. Children with this profile may show insensitivity toward others, a disregard for rules and limits, impulsivity, and hostility. Truly delinquent behavior, such as verbal and physical aggression, destructiveness, lying, and stealing, may be exhibited by some children.

The mean PIC profile of the Internalized Psychopathology subtype (Figure 3.7) displays prominent elevations on a number of subscales that suggest significant internalized socioemotional difficulties. This profile includes high scores on the Adjustment, Depression, Withdrawal, Anxiety, and Psychosis scales, with moderate (though clinically relevant) elevations on Achievement, Development, and Social Skills scales. Children in the Internalized Psychopathology subtype are likely to be depressed, anxious, and emotionally labile. Inappropriate affect, difficulties with cognition and orientation to reality, and social isolation have been associated with this profile. Social interaction and general interpersonal functioning may present serious problems for these children.

The mean PIC profile of the Externalized Psychopathology subtype (Figure 3.8) is also elevated on a number of scales. Children in this subtype have particularly high mean scores on the Adjustment, Delinquency, Hyperactivity, and Social Skills scales. This profile also suggests significant behavioral disturbance; however, unlike children in the Internalized Psychopathology subtype, these children are apt to exhibit hyperkinetic, acting-out types of behavior. Such children may be hostile, impulsive, restless, and emotionally unstable, and may exhibit low frustration tolerance. Aggressive, violent, and destructive behavior may also be part of the clinical picture.

Relations between Age and Psychosocial Functioning

Of the five studies discussed above, the relations between age and patterns of psychosocial functioning were directly examined only in Study 5 (Fuerst & Rourke, 1991b). The results of this investigation seem to suggest that there is no change in the diversity of patterns of psychosocial functioning in children with LD with increasing age. Indeed, there was remarkable stability in patterns of functioning across the age ranges examined in Study 5. No evidence was found to support the notion that children with LD are at risk for the emergence of pathological patterns of psychosocial functioning as they grow older. Similarly, the results of this study indicate that, given a particular pattern of psychosocial adaptation, there is no substantial change in level of adaptation with increasing age. Thus, overall, as children with LD grow older, this study reveals no increased risk for the development of pathological patterns of psychosocial adaptation or any deterioration in level of psychosocial functioning.

These results are very much at variance with Hypothesis 2 formulations of the psychosocial functioning of children with LD (see Chapter 2). Recall that such formulations generally hold that the negative consequences of having LD—such as frustration, anxiety, or peer rejection due to continued academic failure, or a discrete cognitive deficit that perpetually disrupts psychosocial functioning—in time produce maladjustment by grinding down the child's adaptive capacity in some fashion. Although cumulative negative experiences may be deleterious to some children with LD, the results of Study 5 (Fuerst & Rourke, 1991b) and other research (e.g., Chapman, 1988; Chapman & Boersma, 1980; Jorm, Share, Matthews, & Maclean, 1986; and Strang, 1981) suggest strongly that this is not generally the case. It is clear that some children with LD evidence significant maladjustment (e.g., the Internalized Psychopathology and Externalized Psychopathology subtypes); however, the development of pathological patterns of functioning is not more likely with increasing age, nor is deterioration in level of adaptation.

This conclusion must, of course, be tempered by the same consideration that motivated the studies reviewed in this chapter: heterogeneity. Just as some children with LD will not fall neatly within the typology presented above (to the chagrin of statistically oriented researchers, outliers *do* have the annoying habit of showing up in the clinic waiting room), experience dictates that some children with LD demonstrate increasing degrees of abnormal psychosocial development. However, the results of Studies 1 through 5 suggest that when such changes are observed in clinical settings, factors other than simple increased age and cumulative exposure to negative experiences must be considered. An example of a specific, well-delineated subpopulation of children with LD that *does* exhibit exacerbations in abnormal psychosocial development with advancing age, and the factors that may cause or contribute to this process, are presented in the next chapter.

Conclusions

The results of Studies 1 through 5 constitute a formidable, perhaps irrefutable, challenge to the view that children with LD are relatively uniform in terms of their socioemotional functioning. The results of these studies suggest strongly that some children who meet commonly accepted definitions of LD show signs of significant socioemotional disturbance, whereas others do not; on balance, it appears that most do not. Furthermore, these studies cast doubt on the notion that LD, broadly considered, constitute a sufficient condition for the production of emotional disturbance. The important question at this juncture becomes one of determining whether there is a set of characteristics that differentiates (1) children with LD who develop adaptive socioemotional functioning from those children who develop maladaptive socioemotional functioning (i.e., presence or absence of psychopathology, and/or level of psychopathology); and (2) children with LD who develop particular patterns of psychosocial functioning (i.e., different types of pathology, such as internalized vs. externalized). This issue is discussed in greater detail in the next chapter, wherein relations between neuropsychological skill/ability patterns and socioemotional disturbance are examined.

4

Psychosocial Functioning of Children with Learning Disabilities: Review of Hypothesis 3, and Conclusions

HYPOTHESIS 3: Specific Patterns of Central
Processing Abilities and Deficits Cause Specific
Manifestations (Subtypes) of Learning Disabilities and
Specific Forms of Socioemotional Disturbance

Hypothesis 3, the second major hypothesis that has been investigated in this area, proposes a causal connection between particular patterns of central processing abilities and deficits on the one hand, and particular subtypes of both learning disabilities (LD) and socioemotional functioning on the other (Rourke & Fisk, 1981). In other words, deficits in the academic and behavioral adaptation of children with LD are not seen as directly related (except in a correlational sense), as in Hypothesis 2 approaches; instead, both of these sets of difficulties are seen as determined primarily by neurocognitive or neuropsychological strengths and deficiencies.

Methodological and Developmental Considerations

This formulation of the interrelations between patterns of neuropsychological assets and deficits on the one hand, and patterns of

LD and psychosocial functioning on the other, is relatively new. Unfortunately, some of the research in this area has been of less than stellar quality (see Weller & Strawser, 1987, for a brief review of relevant studies). A rather extreme example is found in a study by Stellern, Marlowe, Jacobs, and Cossairt (1985), in which the investigators attempted to relate hemispheric cognitive modes (or styles) to academic performance, classroom behavior, and emotional disturbance in a sample of behavior-disordered and normal control children. Cognitive style (i.e., left hemisphere preferred, right hemisphere preferred, or integrated) was assessed by means of a paper-and-pencil self-report scale. Briefly, Stellern et al. (1985) found that emotional disturbance was weakly associated with a right-hemisphere cognitive mode. In addition to poor subject selection procedures, unsophisticated and questionable statistical methods, and the use of an unvalidated measurement instrument, the entire premise of left- versus right-hemisphere cognitive modes reveals a rather limited and largely erroneous view of brain–behavior relations.

A marginally better study is one by Glosser and Koppell (1987). In this investigation, the authors divided 67 children with learning problems (so identified by referral sources with no other criteria used) into left-hemisphere impairment, right-hemisphere impairment, or nonlateralized impairment. Unfortunately, the classification scheme used was only vaguely described by the authors; it appears to have been developed to provide adequate coverage when the sample was partitioned, rather than rationally or empirically based. The three groups were compared on scores derived from behavioral checklists created by the investigators. Overall, children showing left-hemisphere impairment (as judged by the authors) tended to show more evidence of depression and anxiety, whereas children showing right-hemisphere impairment tended to have more somatic complaints. Those children with nonlateralized impairment tended to show more distractibility, motor activity, and aggression. Roughly comparable results have been reported by Nussbaum and Bigler (1986), who found that children with putative left-hemisphere impairment (judged on the basis of measures of psychometric intelligence and academic achievement) showed somewhat greater levels of personality and behavioral deviance.

More recently, Nussbaum et al. (1988) administered a battery of neuropsychological tests to 219 children from 7 to 12 years old, referred for testing because of learning problems. The investigators developed composite "anterior" and "posterior" cortical impairment scores based on neuropsychological measures used in the assessment. On the basis of these composite scores they classified 33 subjects into either anterior or posterior impairment groups. These two groups were then compared on the Child Behavior Checklist (CBCL; Achenbach & Edelbrock, 1983) and PIC (Wirt, Lachar, Klinedinst, & Seat, 1982), both completed by parents. The results showed that the anterior impairment group showed more evidence of social withdrawal, aggression, hyperactivity, and externalizing pathology, whereas the posterior impairment group showed somewhat greater levels of anxiety.

Although these and other studies fall within the framework of Hypothesis 3 investigations, they clearly represent little or no improvement over many of the Hypothesis 2 investigations reviewed in Chapter 2, for much the same methodological reasons (poor or absent definitions of LD, poor operationalization of psychological constructs, questionable classification procedures, etc.). Disregard of developmental considerations is also of particular concern in these investigations.

There is a tendency in some studies to assume that brain–behavior relations derived from research with adults can be extrapolated without modification to children with LD. For example, it is often assumed that a particular test that may have some value for localization of dysfunction in adults with demonstrated cerebral insult necessarily has similar significance across all age ranges and populations. As Rourke, Bakker, Fisk, and Strang (1983) have pointed out, there are numerous reasons (e.g., rapid maturation of the nervous system, loss of existing ability vs. failure to acquire ability, abnormal or atypical development) why generalization of adult models of cerebral functioning to children must be done with extreme caution and needs to be subjected to careful empirical testing. Similarly, in some studies there is a tendency to frame research problems within static models of limited scope (or, worse still, to present entirely atheoretical investigations). Research undertaken within a limited or trivial theoretical framework tends to produce limited or trivial results. Recent review and theoretical papers by Spreen (1989) and Rourke (1988a, 1988b) have emphasized the need to consider both the components and the dynamics of neurological, cognitive, academic, and psychosocial development and adaptation when developing models to account for the socio-emotional difficulties faced by children with LD. Although this is clearly a monumental task, choosing to ignore complexity when formulating research questions does not make a phenomenon under investigation simpler.

A more sophisticated test of Hypothesis 3 involves an examination of the results of several LD subtype investigations aimed at the determination of patterns of central processing abilities and deficits that characterize such subtypes, and the patterns of socioemotional responsivity that appear to be related to them. We turn now to an analysis of investigations that bear upon these two issues.

Patterns of Central Processing Abilities and Deficits

Regarding the first issue, the results of studies by Rourke and Finlayson (1978), Rourke and Strang (1978), and Strang and Rourke (1983) have demonstrated that 9- to 14-year-old children with LD who exhibit a pattern of impaired reading (word recognition) and spelling within a context of a significantly better, though still impaired, level of performance in mechanical arithmetic (Group R-S) differ markedly in their patterns of neuropsychological abilities and deficits from those who exhibit a pattern of above-average reading and spelling and an outstandingly deficient level of mechanical arithmetic performance (Group A).

As summarized in Strang and Rourke (1985b), these differences cover a wide range of skills and abilities. Specifically, Group A children exhibit below-normal performances on tasks requiring visual–spatial–organizational, psychomotor, tactile–perceptual, and conceptual skills and abilities, within a context of normal performances on verbal tasks that require rote, overlearned verbal skills. They also have difficulties on measures that involve novel task requirements, whether these are "verbal" or "nonverbal" in nature. Group R-S children exhibit virtually the opposite pattern of neuropsychological skills and abilities: mild to moderate difficulties in almost all areas of linguistic endeavor, and marked problems in auditory–perceptual tasks that tax their capacities for exact hearing of speech sounds; normal visual–spatial–organizational, psychomotor, tactile–perceptual, and nonverbal concept formation skills and abilities. In addition, complex problem solving, hypothesis testing, and concept formation in situations where verbal instructions and response requirements are kept to a minimum pose no difficulties for Group R-S children.

This is one group of studies that has demonstrated that subtypes of children formed on the basis of patterns of academic achievement have predictable patterns of neuropsychological assets and deficits. These results have been replicated and expanded in other laboratories (e.g., Fletcher, 1985).

Patterns of Socioemotional Responsivity: Validity Studies

We turn now to a review of studies carried out in our laboratory that have focused on the psychosocial functioning of subtypes of children and adolescents with LD. These studies have their origins in the discovery of the neuropsychological dimensions of the Group R-S and Group A children, and they have followed a course best described as an attempt to develop a nomological net and exploit a form of the multitrait–multimethod approach to validity (Cook & Campbell, 1979). All of these studies bear upon the second issue under immediate consideration—namely, whether and to what extent specific patterns of socioemotional responsivity are related to specific patterns of neuropsychological assets and deficits in children with LD.

The Strang and Rourke (1985a) Study

When the average PIC profiles of children chosen to approximate the characteristics of these two subtypes of children with LD were compared (Strang & Rourke, 1985a), it was clear that the profile for Group A was similar to that exhibited by the "Internalized Psychopathology" group in the Porter and Rourke (1985) and Fuerst, Fisk, and Rourke (1989) studies, whereas the profile for Group R-S children was virtually identical to that exhibited by the "Normal" group in those studies. Additional examination of three factor scores derived from the PIC revealed that Groups R-S and A did not differ significantly on the Concern over Academic Achievement factor, but that they differed sharply on the factors of Personality Deviance and Internalized Psychopathology. In both of the latter cases, the Group A levels of deviation were significantly higher (i.e., more pathological) than were those for Group R-S.

These two sets of results, taken together, offer strong support for Hypothesis 3—namely, that particular patterns of central processing abilities can eventuate in (1) markedly different subtypes of LD (Groups R-S and A) and (2) markedly different patterns of socioemotional functioning (one characterized by normality, the other by an internalized form of psychopathology and personality deviance). Since such group results can be deceiving when applied to the individual case, it should be emphasized that there was very little variance evident in the PIC protocols of the children classified into Groups R-S and A in these studies. Furthermore, the interested reader may wish to consult case studies of such youngsters in three recent works (Rourke, 1989; Rourke et al., 1983; Rourke, Fisk, & Strang, 1986) for evidence of such consistent differences in socioemotional manifestations.

The Fuerst, Fisk, and Rourke (1990) and Fuerst and Rourke (1991a) investigations (reviewed in Chapter 3) also attempted to address Hypothesis 3 considerations. However, in these studies we took the opposite approach to that employed in the Strang and Rourke (1985a) investigation, in that we first attempted to develop a psychosocial typology (using the PIC and statistical methods), and then examined the manner in which these subtypes differed on cognitive and academic measures. The methodological significance of these investigations (i.e., the issue of heterogeneity) has been discussed previously in connection with Hypothesis 2. Our focus here is on the Hypothesis 3 implications of these results.

The Fuerst et al. (1990) Study

In the Fuerst et al. (1990) study, the subjects were selected so as to comprise three (equal-sized) groups with distinctly different patterns of Wechsler Intelligence Scale For Children (WISC; Wechsler, 1949) Verbal IQ (VIQ) and Performance IQ (PIQ) scores. One group had VIQ greater than PIQ by at least 10 points (VIQ > PIQ); a second had VIQ less than PIQ by at least 10 points (VIQ < PIQ); and a third had VIQ and PIQ scores within 9 points of each other (VIQ = PIQ). As discussed earlier (see Chapter 3), the application of several cluster-analytic techniques in this study yielded a reliable solution suggesting the presence of six distinct personality subtypes. The frequencies of the three VIQ–PIQ groups within each of these psychosocial subtype were calculated and compared (see Figure 4.1).

We found that within the Normal subtype, children with VIQ > PIQ occurred at a much lower frequency (roughly 6% of the subtype) than did either children with the opposite pattern (VIQ < PIQ) or those with no significant difference between VIQ and PIQ. This was also the case in the Mild Anxiety subtype, in which subjects with VIQ > PIQ were found at a rate significantly below expectation (about 5% of the subtype). In the Mild Hyperactive subtype, the frequencies of subjects from the three VIQ–PIQ groups were approximately equal. These results indicated that, overall, within normal and mildly disturbed subtypes of children

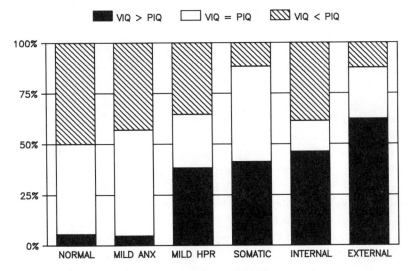

FIGURE 4.1. Proportions of subjects with VIQ > PIQ, VIQ = PIQ, and VIQ <PIQ, in the subtypes developed in the Fuerst, Fisk, and Rourke (1990) study.

with LD, there was a tendency for VIQ > PIQ children to occur at lower frequencies than did VIQ = PIQ or VIQ < PIQ children. There were only about half as many VIQ > PIQ children in these three groups as there were VIQ = PIQ or VIQ < PIQ children.

In the Internalized Psychopathology subtype, subjects with VIQ = PIQ were found at frequencies sig ificantly lower than expected (about 15% of the subtype). On the other hand, subjects with VIQ > PIQ were found at a higher frequency than would be expected (roughly 46% of the subtype), and at a higher frequency than VIQ < PIQ subjects (39%). Within the Externalized Psychopathology subtype, subjects with VIQ > PIQ were found at a much higher frequency (about 63% of the group) than were children with either VIQ = PIQ or VIQ < PIQ. Thus, unlike the normal and mildly disturbed subtypes, subtypes characterized by severe psychosocial disturbance showed a strong tendency to include VIQ > PIQ subjects at higher frequencies than either the VIQ = PIQ or VIQ < PIQ subjects. In total, there were about twice as many VIQ > PIQ children in these two "severe" groups as there were VIQ = PIQ or VIQ < PIQ children.

The Fuerst and Rourke (1991a) Study

In the Fuerst and Rourke (1991a) investigation, six personality subtypes were also generated (see Chapter 3). With one exception, these were the same subtypes as those found in the Fuerst et al. (1990) study. The differences among these six subtypes on Wide Range Achievement Test (WRAT; Jastak & Jastak, 1965) Reading, Spelling, and Arithmetic standard scores were examined (see Figure 4.2). Overall, the six subtypes were indiscriminable on WRAT Arithmetic. However, there were significant differences among some of the subtypes on WRAT Reading and Spelling. The Externalized Psychopathology and Internalized Psychopathology subtypes had mean WRAT Reading scores that were significantly higher than those of the Somatic Concern and Normal subtypes. Similarly, the Externalized and Internalized Psychopathology subtypes scored higher on WRAT Spelling than did the Conduct Disorder and Normal groups, and the Internalized Psychopathology group also scored higher than did the Somatic Concern group.

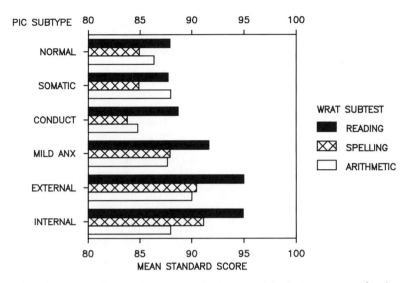

FIGURE 4.2. Mean WRAT Reading, Spelling, and Arithmetic scores for the subtypes found in the Fuerst and Rourke (1991a) study.

These findings were echoed when WRAT Reading, Spelling, and Arithmetic were considered simultaneously in a canonical discriminant analysis. The first canonical function was significant, providing better than chance discrimination between the groups. When the standardized scoring coefficients for this function were considered, it was apparent that scores on this variable were virtually simple sums of WRAT Reading and Spelling scores (i.e., these scores had approximately equal weights), with Arithmetic playing a trivial role. Examination of group means on the canonical variables indicated that the Normal, Somatic Concern, and Conduct Disorder groups were indistinguishable on this variable. These three groups were, however, clearly separated from the higher-scoring Externalized and Internalized Psychopathology groups, which appeared to form a second "clump" on their own. The Mild Anxiety group fell about midway between these two sets of subtypes.

These results suggest that children with relatively well-developed reading (word recognition) and spelling skills are more likely to appear in PIC subtypes with profiles suggestive of severe psychopathology, be it of the internalizing or externalizing type. On the other hand, children with relatively mild somatization or conduct disorder problems are indistinguishable from normal children on the basis of reading and spelling skills. Children with symptoms of mild anxiety and depression appear to fall between these two extremes, and cannot be distinguished from either on the basis of these skills.

We (Fuerst & Rourke, 1991a) also compared the groups on differences in WRAT Reading minus Arithmetic and Spelling minus Arithmetic scores. Overall, the Internalized Psychopathology group showed not only the largest absolute difference on these two measures, but also showed deficient Arithmetic relative to both Reading and Spelling (i.e., a pattern identical to that shown by the Group A subtype in previous studies). Specifically, on the Reading minus Arithmetic measure, the Internalized Psychopathology group was significantly different from the Somatic Concern group; on the Spelling minus Arithmetic measure, they were significantly different from the Normal group. None of the other subtypes could be differentiated on either Reading minus Arithmetic or Spelling minus Arithmetic.

Implications

Although the results of these studies are quite straightforward, the patterns of relations revealed by the studies and the implications of these patterns are fairly complex and require detailed explanation, as follows.

1. Strang and Rourke (1985a) demonstrated that Group A subjects (good reading and spelling relative to arithmetic) evidence more psychopathology of clinical significance than do Group R-S subjects (poor reading and spelling relative to arithmetic). We (Fuerst & Rourke, 1991a) also demonstrated that children evidencing severe psychopathology tend to perform better in reading and spelling than do children with normal psychosocial functioning or relatively benign psychosocial problems. Both the Strang and Rourke (1985a) and Fuerst and Rourke (1991a) studies also revealed that children showing a Group A pattern of academic performance tend to evidence a particular *type* of psychopathology (internalized).

Thus, there is a relationship between patterns of academic functioning and patterns of psychosocial functioning (both level and type of pathology) in children with LD.

2. It is difficult to argue that patterns of academic performance (i.e., good reading and spelling relative to arithmetic, or vice versa) influence psychosocial functioning. That is, there is no obvious explanation for the observation that Group A children evidence greater psychopathology than do Group R-S children. Similarly, it is also difficult to argue that different patterns of psychosocial functioning can directly produce different patterns of academic achievement. (An exception to this assertion might be cases of primary psychopathology, such as major depressive disorder or attention deficit disorder. As explained in the discussion of Hypothesis 1 in Chapter 2, these cases lie outside the realm of LD.)

3. In regard to point 2, it is logical to propose that there is a third factor accounting for the apparent relationship between patterns of academic functioning and psychosocial functioning. Although it is certainly possible that there could be many different factors producing this apparent relationship, a single factor would provide the most parsimonious explanation.

4. The most likely candidate for this intervening factor is cognitive functioning. Previous research has clearly indicated that patterns of academic functioning are strongly related to patterns of cognitive functioning, as measured by neuropsychological/psychometric instruments. These measures include, but are by no means limited to, WISC VIQ–PIQ discrepancies (Rourke, Dietrich, & Young, 1973; Rourke & Finlayson, 1978; Rourke & Telegdy, 1971; Rourke, Young, & Flewelling, 1971). The logical direction of causation in this relationship is that cognitive factors influence academic performance.

5. The Fuerst et al. (1990) results have demonstrated that patterns of cognitive functioning, measured by WISC VIQ–PIQ discrepancy, are associated with psychosocial functioning. Specifically, children showing the pattern of WISC VIQ > PIQ tend to be found in subtypes demonstrating severe psychopathology, whereas children with VIQ = PIQ or VIQ < PIQ tend to be found in subtypes with normal or mildly disturbed psychosocial functioning. As before, it is difficult to conceive of patterns of psychosocial function-

ing as causing patterns of cognitive functioning (with the exceptions noted above). It is more logical to propose that patterns of cognitive functioning influence psychosocial functioning.

6. Thus, it follows that cognitive–neuropsychological functioning may, at one and the same time, influence academic performance on the one hand and psychosocial functioning on the other. Patterns of cognitive–neuropsychological functioning may be the intervening factors accounting for the apparent relationship between academic performance and socioemotional adjustment. However, further investigation, using more direct and detailed measures of cognitive and neuropsychological functioning, is required in order to have greater confidence in this conclusion.

Other Studies

Two investigations that were designed to determine the developmental outcome for Group A children are also useful for evaluating Hypothesis 3. Rourke, Young, Strang, and Russell (1986) compared the performances of Group A children and a group of clinic-referred adults on a wide variety of neuropsychological variables. The adults presented with VIQ–PIQ discrepancies and WRAT patterns that were virtually identical to the analogous patterns in Group A children. It was demonstrated that the patterns of age-related performances of the adults and the children on the neuropsychological variables were remarkably similar. In addition, the adults were characterized by internalized forms of psychopathology that bore a striking resemblance to those exhibited by Group A youngsters. In a related study, Del Dotto, Rourke, McFadden, and Fisk (1987) confirmed the stability of the neuropsychological and personality characteristics of this subtype of persons with LD over time.

It should also be noted that Weintraub and Mesulam (1983) have described the socioemotional, cognitive, and neurological status of 14 adults who were very similar to the Group A subtype. The patients showed neurological abnormalities; large discrepancies (as much as 36 points) between VIQ and PIQ in favor of the latter (with the exception of one case); poor memory for nonverbal material relative to verbal material; poor eye contact in interview; and reduced speech prosody. Chronic shyness, introversion, social isolation, and depression were very common in the sample. Denckla (1983) has also reported clinical experiences consistent with those of Weintraub and Mesulam (1983).

Finally, a series of investigations by Tramontana and colleagues, while not of direct relevance to the psychosocial functioning of children with LD, are of some interest in this context. In an early study, Tramontana, Sherrets, and Golden (1980) examined the neuropsychological performance of 20 psychiatric patients between 9 and 15 years of age, who had no history of neuropathological conditions or positive neurological findings. Overall, some 60% of subjects demonstrated neuropsychological impairment; of those subjects, 25% performed as poorly as would frankly brain-injured patients be expected to perform. Difficulties with reading, spelling, and complex perceptual and problem-solving tasks were most common. A later study by Tramontana and Sherrets (1985) with a similar sample produced essentially the same results: About 50% of children with frank psychopathology also demonstrated significantly impaired neuropsychological test results. In addition, Tramontana and Sherrets (1985) found that subjects showing impaired neuropsychological performance also had anomalous computed tomography (CT) results relative to unimpaired subjects (although, in the absence of suitable controls, the CT findings for impaired subjects were not necessarily abnormal). More recently, Tramontana, Hooper, and Nardolillo (1988) found that, in young (8–11 years of age) male psychiatric patients, neuropsychological impairment was associated with more extensive behavior problems, especially of the internalizing type.

Of course, impaired performance on neuropsychological tests does not necessarily signify impairment in cognitive functions thought to be tapped by those measures, or disruption in neural substrates that may be associated with those functions. Unusual motivational and/or behavioral factors associated with significant psychopathology can also influence performance on neuropsychological tests, creating an inflated false-positive rate of impairment in psychiatric samples. (This issue and others that complicate the interpretation of neuropsychological results in a psychiatric context are discussed in Tramontana, 1983.) Furthermore, the studies by Tramontana and colleagues also suffer from many of the methodological problems discussed above (including lack of a theoretical framework and failure to account for heterogeneity). However, in the context of the studies reviewed in the previous section, these findings offer some support for the contention that psychosocial and cognitive functioning are associated in children. The extent to which facets of that association are predictable and of clinical import in children with frank psychopathology is not yet known.

Summary

It would appear that children who exhibit the Group A (nonverbal learning disabilities, or NLD) profile of neuropsychological abilities and deficits are likely to be described by parents as emotionally or behaviorally disturbed. In contrast, Group R-S children (with outstanding difficulties in many aspects of psycholinguistic functioning) are so described at much lower frequencies. More generally, it may be that the Group A pattern of NLD is a sufficient condition for the development of some sort of socioemotional disturbance (Rourke, 1987, 1988b, 1989), whereas the pattern of central processing abilities and deficits exhibited by the Group R-S subtype examined in this series of studies may not constitute the same sufficient basis for such an outcome.

This is not meant to imply that children characterized by the Group R-S (language-deficient) pattern will never experience socioemotional disturbance. Indeed, clinical experience (e.g., Rourke et al., 1983; Rourke, Fisk, & Strang, 1986) suggests that many do. Rather, these results suggest that, for the Group R-S subtype, factors in addition to psycholinguistic deficiency may be necessary for disturbed socioemotional functioning to occur. Such additional factors may include some of those mentioned in connection with the emotional disturbance–learning problem relationship outlined in Chapter 2 of this book (e.g., teacher–pupil personality conflicts, unrealistic demands by parents and teachers, and inappropriate motivation and social expectancies). Others would appear to include the presence of salient antisocial models, selective reinforcement of nonadaptive and socially inappropriate behaviors, and any number of other factors that have the potential for encouraging problems in the socioemotional functioning of even normally achieving youngsters.

Refinements of these findings and detailed theoretical explanations of their interrelations are contained in several recent publications (e.g., Rourke, 1982, 1987, 1989, 1991; Rourke & Fisk, 1988; Strang & Rourke, 1985a). Although it is relatively easy to demonstrate and outline this pattern of relations, as we have done in the "Implications" section above, the development and articulation of a model capable of accounting for those relations is a far more complex undertaking. A detailed model that accounts for the propensity of the child with NLD to develop a particular configuration of academic learning difficulties and a specific type of severe socioemotional disturbance (plus many other unusual features often noted by clinicians when dealing with such children) is presented in Rourke (1989) and summarized in Rourke, Del Dotto, Rourke, and Casey (1990). The critical features of this model are also discussed in Chapter 5, wherein we present two examples of children with the NLD syndrome.

Briefly, and at the risk of oversimplification, these tendencies of the child with NLD have been characterized in terms of the development of, and interaction between, deficits in primary (e.g., basic perceptual and motor skills), secondary (e.g., attention to stimuli in various modalities), and tertiary (e.g., mnestic, concept formation, and problem-solving abilities) neuropsychological functions. Well-developed processing capacities within auditory–verbal domains, together with poor capacity within perceptual–motor, concept formation, problem-solving, and other nonverbal domains, are seen as resulting in the development of good rote reading and spelling skills but pronounced difficulty with mechanical arithmetic. Given deficits in nonverbal skills, and difficulty in dealing with complex or novel situations, but relative strengths in many aspects of psycholinguistic abilities, these children also come to rely excessively on rote auditory–verbal skills for interacting with others. As a result, children with NLD tend to misperceive/mis-emit, or simply miss/fail to emit, most of the subtle and not-so-subtle nonverbal information in their interchanges with others. These children also lack the capacity to deal effectively with the complex and novel problems that inevitably arise in dealing with others. As a result, they tend to have grave problems in interpersonal relations. As they grow older, and the demands of interpersonal relationships become more complex and the price of failure higher, they tend to become socially isolated and withdrawn. Concurrently, their academic problems also become more pronounced, as they are faced with the much more complex demands of secondary and postsecondary education—demands that their circumscribed strengths in rote verbal abilities cannot meet. In consequence, their educational/vocational outlook becomes quite poor. Their psychosocial adaptation deteriorates, and pronounced internalized psychopathology often becomes evident.

Empirical evidence consistent with this model, summarized in Rourke (1989, 1991), has been growing very rapidly. In the most recent study, Casey, Rourke, and Picard (1991) contrasted the psychosocial functioning of samples of younger (about 8 years of age) and older (about 13 years) children that met criteria for NLD. They found that the mean PIC profiles exhibited by both groups were very similar to the prototypical Internalized Psychopathology profile derived from the Windsor taxonomic research. However, the mean PIC profile of the older children was clearly more deviant than that of the younger children, with an extreme score on the Psychosis scale (greater than 90 T), and significant elevations on the Depression and Social Skills scales. Overall, the PIC profile of the older children with NLD was more elevated (i.e., more disturbed), especially on scales related to internalized psychopathology. Thus, although children with LD may in general show no apparent predisposition for increased psychopathology with advancing age, a specific subpopulation of children—those with NLD—is at risk for the development of significant psychopathology (of the internalizing kind) with increasing age.

The actual model presented by Rourke (1989) is much more complex than this brief synopsis. The dynamic interplay and development of the components within the model are further cast upon a foundation of empirical and theoretical models of central nervous system development in children. Thus, the model is also capable of encompassing some of the complex manifestations of specific neuropathological conditions (such as head injury, extensive radiotherapy of the central nervous system, and neurotoxic conditions) that are likely to produce the NLD syndrome. At the same time, it is clear that the etiologies of NLD are by no means limited to frank cerebral insult. Although there is a good fit between the model and clinical experience, and empirical evidence is rapidly mounting to support it (the most recent of which is presented in Rourke, 1991), further research is required to test many aspects of the model.

CONCLUSIONS

Principal Conclusions

Clearly, our understanding of the psychosocial development and functioning of children with LD is far from complete. However, our review of the available literature in this and the foregoing chapters suggests that, although many studies have been less informative than might be hoped, research efforts in this area have not been wasted. The conclusions that flow from our review of this literature are as follows:

1. There is no single, unitary pattern of personality characteristics, psychosocial adaptation, social competence, self-concept, locus of control, or other facet of socioemotional functioning that is characteristic of all children with LD.

2. Some children with LD experience mild to severe disturbance of socioemotional functioning. However, most children with LD appear to achieve adequate psychosocial adaptation.

3. There are distinct types of socioemotional disturbance and behavior disorder that may be displayed by children with LD. These various manifestations of emotional and behavioral disorder may be somewhat more frequent among children with LD than among their normally achieving peers; however, the precise types and incidence of emotional and behavioral problems in children with LD are as yet not known.

4. One pattern of central processing abilities and deficits (NLD) appears to lead to a particular configuration of academic achievement (well-developed word recognition and spelling, as compared to significantly poorer mechanical arithmetic), increased risk of psychopathology, and a tendency to develop an internalized form of socioemotional disturbance. Other patterns of central processing abilities and deficits (those marked by outstanding difficulties in psycholinguistic skills) appear to lead to particular patterns of academic achievement (striking problems in reading and spelling; varying levels of performance in mechanical arithmetic), with

some correlative effect upon the incidence of psychopathology, but with no particular effect upon its specific manifestations.

5. There is no conclusive evidence that children with LD are more susceptible than are their normally achieving peers to problems with substance abuse, truly antisocial behavior, or delinquency. Carefully conducted longitudinal research suggests that, as a group, children with LD are no more likely to develop these problems than are normal children.

6. There is no conclusive evidence that children with LD as a group tend to become more susceptible to socioemotional disturbance with advancing age, relative to normally achieving peers.

7. One exception to point 6 is the worsening in the manifestations of psychopathology and the increasing discrepancies between abilities and deficits that are exhibited by children and adolescents with NLD. This is the case in spite of the fact that the pattern of neuropsychological abilities and deficits and the specific manifestations of psychopathology in such individuals remain quite stable over time.

Clinical Generalizations and Conclusions

General Observations

Some children, adolescents, and adults experience socioemotional problems that prevent progress in learning in school and elsewhere. It is important to direct treatment at the socioemotional disturbances exhibited by such individuals. The following are some general observations and guidelines that may help to direct such efforts:

1. In the case of persons whose learning problems are caused by socioemotional disturbance, one would expect that once this disturbance is treated effectively (especially if it is treated at an early age), learning will proceed apace.

2. In the case of individuals whose psychosocial difficulties are (largely or in part) the direct result of, or strongly linked to, their LD, it is necessary to direct therapeutic attention in some systematic way to both of these sets of problems.

3. For persons whose LD and socioemotional difficulties result from a common cause (e.g., some form of central processing abili-

ties and deficits), clinicians should attempt to (a) ameliorate those basic central processing deficits that are amenable to change, and (b) provide compensatory coping strategies and techniques for those deficits that are not likely to change.

Clinical Conclusions

The following are some clinical conclusions arising from this review of the literature that should be made quite explicit:

1. The social status of persons with LD would appear to be an important dimension relating to their feelings of well-being and their level of psychosocial functioning. It appears that some children and adolescents with LD have lower social status (in the judgment of others) than do their normally achieving peers. However, the variance in this dimension exhibited by children and adolescents with LD (i.e., ranging from well below average to well above average) would suggest strongly that the presence of LD is not an unambiguous marker for level of social status. Hence, if clinically justified, a specific determination of the social status of the person with LD should be carried out in conjunction with other assessment methods. Failure to measure such a dimension explicitly may limit the understanding of the clinician and, in turn, may jeopardize the treatment of the person with LD.

2. The evidence relating self-esteem to LD is equivocal. Among other things, this would suggest that the person with LD who presents with significant deficits in self-esteem may not be suffering from such problems as a result of deficits in learning within the academic milieu. Rather, it is much more probable that, in such a case, problems in self-esteem have a separate etiology quite apart from the LD. Hence, a coordinated therapeutic program that takes into consideration the essentially unrelated nature of each of these sets of disorders is likely to be most effective.

3. Learned helplessness may be exhibited by some children and adolescents with LD. However, in this instance as well, it is quite probable that such dimensions of "problem" behavior are the result of etiological factors that are not directly attributable to LD per se. Hence, treatment will, in all probability, be directed at changing learned helplessness without particular regard to the person's LD.

4. The absence of any apparent relationship between advancing years and degree of psychosocial disturbance in children and adolescents with LD should not be taken to imply that early intervention with such persons is not desirable. The apparent absence of significant age-related changes in these important dimensions of behavior may reflect the operation of compensatory behaviors that are, in the long run, of unknown desirability. In any case, significant socioemotional disturbance should be treated without regard to data suggesting that such disturbance does not increase with age.

5. Every clinician aims to treat patients on an individualized basis. However, there is something to be gained from taking into consideration the notion of subtypes, both with respect to LD per se and with respect to the psychosocial problems and difficulties that may accompany them, be caused by them, or arise from a similar or identical source as do the LD themselves. Several dimensions of the subtype issue should be mentioned within this context. These issues have been outlined before (Rourke, 1985), and the earlier statement is presented here as a general formulation of this rather complex problem:

> The classification of children into "homogeneous" subtypes does not imply that the children so classified are identical. Indeed, it would appear quite likely that children classified [into subtypes] . . . would exhibit, together with their similarities, fairly substantial individual differences. That is, although they may be quite similar to one another with respect to their pattern of adaptive abilities and deficits (and, by implication, with respect to their central processing characteristics), any number of differences in early or current environmental circumstances, reinforcement patterns, and so on would be expected to have a differential impact on the psychosocial functioning of the children. It is for this reason that predictions (prognoses) and treatments must be framed and designed as individual amalgams reflecting common (subtypal) and unique (historical) characteristics.
>
> In this connection, it should be borne in mind that the common (subtypal) variance is itself a reflection of a certain level of uniqueness or individuality, insofar as it differentiates each child within a particular subtype from those in other subtypes and from those who are not classified. In addition, the idiographic formulation of the treatment plan should take into consideration the final level of individualization that is afforded by an examination and understanding of a child's unique sociohistori-

cal milieu and characteristics. It is in this (combined) sense that we view the identification of more general clusters of learning-disabled children who share common dimensions or factors as a complementary form of individualization that (we hope) contributes to the formulation and execution of appropriate individual education/therapeutic plans (Fisk & Rourke, 1983; Rourke, Bakker, Fisk, & Strang, 1983, p. 12). (Rourke, 1985, p. 12)

5

Case Studies

INTRODUCTION

In this chapter we present nine case studies. These cases are designed to illustrate some of the ways in which various patterns of neuropsychological assets and deficits are related to academic and psychosocial difficulties. Although there is an emphasis on case examples of children whose academic learning and psychosocial problems are related to their particular patterns of neuropsychological assets and deficits, cases where this relationship is tenuous or nonexistent are also examined.

We have included seven cases that span the years from early childhood to middle adolescence, and two cases of adults, one of whom was followed over a 14-year period. The adults are included to demonstrate that learning disabilities (LD) can persist into adulthood, and that the interactions between particular patterns of neuropsychological assets and deficits have a predictable relationship to academic and psychosocial functioning in adults as well as in children. The longitudinal follow-ups provided in two cases (Cases 4 and 9) also demonstrate the manner in which such relationships can be seen to follow a predictable course.

The format for the presentation of the cases begins with a statement of the relevance of the case. This is followed by a summary of neuropsychological assessment findings. Most of the assessment findings are couched in a quasi-report format. One of our purposes in these instances is to describe in verbal detail the data that are spread in the figure (which includes a graphic display of the quantitative information gleaned from the examination) that accompanies each case. More important, however, is our purpose of describing in some detail the specific assets and deficits exhibited by each person, and the interactions among and between these that have relevance for academic and psychosocial functioning.

Readers not familiar with the tests employed in our routine neuropsychological examination should consult the Appendix of Rourke (1989), or Rourke, Fisk, and Strang (1986). The latter work (see especially Chs. 1 and 2) also contains details dealing with the approach and rationale of the treatment-oriented neuropsychological assessment that we employ in such cases.

A note about format is in order. The figures that accompany these cases have been designed to illustrate the results of our examination of each individual in quantitative terms. The data have been transformed to T scores based on the age-appropriate norms for each test. In this way, comparability between tests can be determined. For example, a T score of 40 on the Target Test would indicate that the person's score on this test fell exactly one standard deviation below the age-appropriate mean for this test; similarly, a T score of 60 on this test would indicate that this person's score was exactly one standard deviation above the mean for this test. As a result of the use of this norm-referenced metric for each test, all of the scores that are spread in the figure can be compared and contrasted with one another. Note that in some instances there may seem to be minor disagreements between the text and the figures. These apparent discrepancies may arise because the figures present only a subset of the measures available from the complete neuropsychological protocols on which the text is based.

CASE 1: JOHN

Relevance

John is a good example of a child in the early stages of adolescence (11 years, 9 months of age) who is best described as (1) having a subtype of LD we have defined elsewhere as the "output" variety (see Rourke, 1989, Ch. 8, for a description of this subtype), and (2) exhibiting a significant socioemotional disorder, primarily of the "externalized" variety.

His neuropsychological deficits are quite clear: His verbal fluency to rule is very poor. Although John's fund of verbal information may be quite good, he is not able to tap it with any degree of ease. He does not appear to code experiences in a verbal fashion, thus rendering their recall quite problematic. These deficits in the more "expressive" aspects of language would appear to account for his problems in directing his behavior via verbal means, thus rendering the smooth orchestration of his behavior very difficult. Within the academic sphere, virtually all areas of functioning are affected adversely by this set of problems. In much the same vein, his psychosocial functioning is characterized by what many of his caretakers describe as "impulsive" responding.

With respect to the interaction among John's learning difficulties, his academic problems, and his psychosocial difficulties, it would appear fairly clear that the neuropsychological assets and deficits that define his form of LD also lie at the roots of both his academic and psychosocial problems. For example, his "impulsivity" would appear to result from his virtual inability to direct his behavior by verbal means: Rather than considering alternatives or having immediate access to rules governing behavior (both of which require verbal mediation), he turns to action. And these actions are often inappropriate. Within the academic sphere, it is clear that his difficulties in generating verbal answers to questions—especially those that require recall rather than mere recognition of information—are hampering his progress to a significant degree.

It is notable that John's psychosocial behavior and academic performance have begun to improve considerably with the introduction of a multifaceted treatment program that includes use of the modified Think Aloud program (Camp & Bash, 1981); considerable one-to-one tutoring; and encouragements to verbalize what he is doing, what he has just done, and what he is about to do. All of these therapeutic techniques have in common the encouragement of the verbal mediation of behavior—a skill that can be learned to a considerable extent, even by children of this fairly advanced age and with this subtype of LD.

The following are essential elements of the report on John's neuropsychological assessment. Emphasis is placed upon the delineation of his assets and deficits, with a view to demonstrating how these interact to play a role in his academic and social difficulties.

Neuropsychological Assessment Findings

Behavioral Observations during the Examination

Throughout the day-long testing session, John was most uncooperative with the examiner, and rapport was very difficult to obtain and maintain with him. He was quite careless and impulsive on occasion, and rather antagonistic toward the examiner. His general level of psychomotor coordination appeared well developed. He exhibited a below-average amount of verbal interchange with the examiner. There were many occasions when he required considerable encouragement from the examiner to proceed with the tasks at hand. Very often, he exhibited a rather low level of tolerance for frustration. In general, his approach to the tasks presented to him was quite careless; his level of motivation was quite variable. It was apparent that much of the untoward behavior exhibited in this examination was a reaction to his perceived failures on some tests. He also exhibited a rather low level of self-esteem.

All things considered, it would appear that a very reliable estimate of this boy's adaptive skills and abilities was not obtained in this examination. It is apparent that some good performances were elicited in a number of areas, and that some of his poor levels of performance are clearly lower-bound estimates of his skills and abilities in some areas.

Summary of Test Results and Impressions

General Comments. John exhibited some very well-developed skills and abilities. Most of these were evident on tests that did not require much effortful processing of information or much in the way of orchestrated output. However, there were some very clear exceptions to this generalization. There were some apparently reliable deficits in evidence that may indicate more than ordinary difficulties in a variety of forms of expression and the smooth orchestration of behavior. It is clear that his current difficulties would be expected to hamper his attempts at adaptation, especially as regards progress within the academic realm. This situation may be further complicated by his apparently significant difficulties in socioemotional functioning, especially of the externalized variety. The following report was designed to add some specifications to these generalizations and to suggest some avenues to pursue in remedial programming for him. Figure 5.1 provides a summary of John's test scores.*

Test Results and Impressions. There were no indications of any simple tactile imperception with either hand; there was some tactile suppression exhibited with the left hand. John experienced very marked difficulties in identifying symbols written on the fingertips of both hands. There was some evidence of finger agnosia with both hands. He exhibited some difficulties in identifying coins placed within both hands; this was especially marked with the left hand.

On a complex nonverbal problem-solving task (Tactual Performance Test, involving strategy generation, psychomotor coordination, and the capacity to benefit from tactile input and kinesthetic feedback), his levels of performance with each hand separately and

---

*In this and subsequent figures, abbreviations for the PIC profiles are the same as those for figures in Chapter 3. Abbreviations for the histograms are as follows: CATTOT, Category Test, total errors; TRAILSA, Trail Making Test, Part A, time; TRAILSB, Trail Making Test, Part B, time; TPTDT, Tactual Performance Test (TPT), dominant-hand time; TPTNDT, TPT, nondominant-hand time; TPTBT, TPT, both-hands time; TPTTOT, TPT, total time; TPTMEM, TPT, memory; TPTLOC, TPT, location; TARGET, Target Test; SPCHPER, Speech-Sounds Perception Test; AUDCLO, Auditory Closure Test; SENMEM, Sentence Memory Test; FLUENCY, Verbal Fluency Test; APHASIA, total errors on the Aphasia Screening Test; GRIP, dynamometer (strength); TAPPING, finger tapping; NAME, name writing; HOLEST, Graduated Holes Test, time; HOLESC, Graduated Holes Test, contact; MAZEST, Maze Test, time; MAZESC, Maze Test, contact; PEGS, Grooved Pegboard Test; TACSUP, tactile suppression; FAGNOS, finger agnosia; FWRIT, fingertip number writing; TACFORM, tactile forms recognition; AUDSUP, auditory suppression; VISSUP, visual suppression. In the tabular parts of all figures, WISC-R VIQ, PIQ, and FSIQ scores, and PPVT IQ scores, are reported in the usual metric. Scores on the WISC-R subtests are reported as subtest scaled scores. WRAT-R Reading, Spelling, and Arithmetic measures are reported as standard scores (grade-equivalent and centile scores are provided in the text).

with both hands together were markedly impaired. His incidental memory for the shapes and locations of the blocks used on this task was also quite poor. It is very probable that his best possible level of performance was not obtained on this task.

John would appear to be predominantly left-handed, and exclusively right-footed and left-eyed. Strength of grip with both hands was below average, and not in the expected relationship for a left-handed individual. Finger-tapping speed with the left hand was mildly impaired; that with the right, average. He performed below normal limits, especially with the left foot, on a test for foot-tapping speed. His performance on tests specifically designed for the measurement of static and kinetic tremor could not be evaluated with any confidence because of his lack of cooperation in following task instructions. Performance on a test of speeded eye–hand coordination (Grooved Pegboard Test) was superior with the right hand and clearly impaired with the left hand. The inconsistencies noted in these motor and psychomotor tests render performance on them difficult to determine. However, there was rather clear evidence of more impairment in performance with the left hand than with the right hand.

There were no indications of any simple visual imperception or suppression. He performed within normal limits on a test requiring immediate memory for visual sequences (Target Test).

John's graphic renderings of simple visual designs were mildly deficient in terms of their visual–spatial configurations; all were marked by some evidence of tremor. His printing and cursive script were somewhat uncoordinated. His drawing of a complex key was quite immature and lacking in visual–spatial detail; there were also some distortions of visual–spatial detail in evidence. It is probable that some of his difficulties in graphomotor skills relate to problems in guiding his behavior by verbal means.

On a task that requires the use of a pencil and the rendering of fine visual discriminations under timed conditions (Underlining Test), he experienced some difficulty on some of the subtests that involve dealing with sequenced material. However, his performances on others were within the normal to very superior range. His performances on approximately half of the subtests were within normal limits. It is clear that he did not cooperate fully on this test. It is also clear that he is capable of extremely proficient levels of performance when he remains on task.

FIGURE 5.1. Summary of neuropsychological test results for Case 1 (John). Note that *T* scores with a value of 10 or less have been plotted with a value of 10. Measures with missing values have been assigned a *T* score of 0 (i.e., a bar height of 0).

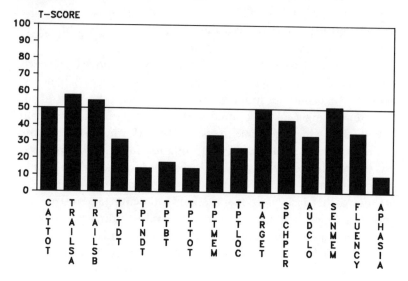

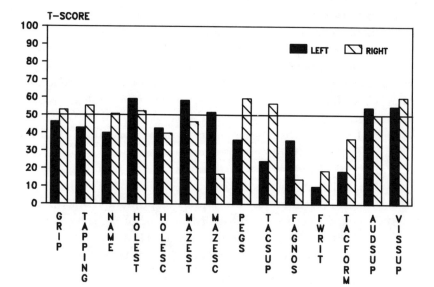

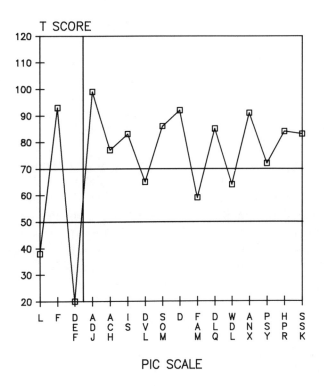

PIC SCALE

Test	Score at 11 yr, 9 mo
WISC-R	
Verbal IQ	84
Information	6
Comprehension	8
Arithmetic	8
Similarities	6
Vocabulary	9
Digit Span	7
Performance IQ	91
Picture Completion	7
Picture Arrangement	12
Block Design	8
Object Assembly	8
Coding	9
Full Scale IQ	86
PPVT IQ	102
WRAT-R	
Reading	67
Spelling	75
Arithmetic	73

On the Performance section of the Wechsler Intelligence Scale for Children—Revised (WISC-R), John obtained a Performance IQ (PIQ) of 91. Subtest scaled scores on this section of the WISC-R ranged from a low of 7 on the Picture Completion subtest to a high of 12 on the Picture Arrangement subtest. It is apparent that John's best possible performances were not obtained on many of these subtests.

His performance was superior on a task that required him to negotiate a visual–spatial array with a pencil on the basis of the numeric sequence (Trail Making Test). When this test was rendered somewhat more complex by the addition of the requirement to alternate between the numeric and alphabetic sequences in order to complete the task, his level of performance was high-average.

There were no indications of any simple auditory imperception or suppression with either ear. Performance on a Sweep Hearing Test was within normal limits. He exhibited a markedly impaired level of performance on a task requiring fine auditory discrimination and sustained attentional skills (Seashore Rhythm Test). It is probable that the sustained attentional requirements of this task were problematic for him.

John performed at a mildly impaired level on a test for sound blending. His performance on a phonemically cued test of verbal fluency was also mildly impaired. A test for verbatim sentence memory was performed at an average level. Performance on a test that required him to underline the graphic equivalents of novel speech sounds was at a borderline level. It is notable that his performances on the final sections of the latter test were flawless.

On the Verbal section of the WISC-R, he obtained a Verbal IQ (VIQ) of 84. Subtest scaled scores on this section of the WISC-R ranged from lows of 6 on the Information and Similarities subtests to a high of 9 on the Vocabulary subtest. This pattern of scores on the WISC-R is most unusual and probably reflects uneven motivation and cooperation during the administration of these subtests. There is no doubt that the VIQ is an underestimate of his general level of psycholinguistic skill development.

On the Peabody Picture Vocabulary Test (PPVT), John obtained a Mental Age of 12 years, 3 months, which is equivalent to an IQ of 102.

On the Aphasia Screening Test, he exhibited difficulty with the following: the oral and written spelling of age-appropriate words;

naming simple figures; enunciation of complex multisyllabic words; simple arithmetic calculation. It is notable that he did not make any significant errors in reading on this test. It is probable that some of his errors on this test were the result of rather impulsive responding.

Performance on a very complex nonverbal problem-solving task (the Category Test, involving concept formation, strategy generation, and the capacity to benefit from positive and negative informational feedback) was within normal limits. This level of performance was attained in spite of John's initial problems in dealing with some of the task requirements and his uneven level of cooperation throughout the test.

On the Wide Range Achievement Test—Revised (WRAT-R), John obtained the following approximate grade-equivalent (centile) scores: Reading, 2 (1); Spelling, 3 (5); Arithmetic, 3 (4). Many of his misspellings of the words on this subtest were of the phonetically inaccurate variety. This may have resulted, in the main, from his impulsive response style. On the Reading subtest, he appeared able to use a phonetic word attack strategy for the decoding of unfamiliar words. However, he seemed to prefer the "sight-word/best-guess" approach (e.g., "sure" for "sour," "stake" for "stalk," "block" for "bulk"). His performance on the Arithmetic subtest suggests that he has mastered most of the principles relating to very basic arithmetic calculation skills; however, his application of these was marked by some carelessness and inattention to detail. In addition, some of his responses were quite bizarre.

On the Personality Inventory for Children (PIC; completed by his father), there were clear indications that this boy is perceived as suffering from a marked degree of socioemotional disturbance (predominantly of the externalized variety). There were similarly clear suggestions of externalized psychopathology evident on a behavior rating scale and on an activity rating scale (also completed by the father).

Neuropsychological Disposition and Implications

This particular pattern of neuropsychological test results would not tend to raise any serious question regarding the functional integrity of John's brain. The clinical picture is one that is compatible with long-standing conduct and/or attention deficit disorder, with possible complications relating to the planning and orchestrating of behavioral strategies. The direction of behavior by verbal means—especially in the absence of corrective feedback—appears to be particularly troublesome for this boy. The latter difficulties might tend to raise some question regarding the functional integrity of the anterior regions of the brain, but the evidence in support of such an assertion is not completely compelling.

John would be expected to experience considerable difficulty in attempting to learn and perform within any number of formal and informal situations. His general problems in the smooth orchestration of behavior and in directing his behavior through verbal means would be expected to hamper his progress in school and in social situations, which, with increasing years, will become much more complex in terms of behavioral demands. In addition, his difficulties in socioemotional adaptation may very well reflect problems in handling what would appear to be continuing experiences of academic failure.

The long-range prognosis for some habilitation of this boy's neuropsychological deficits would appear to be fair. With intensive, specialized intervention at this time, there is some reason to believe that advancement in his adaptive skills and abilities is indeed probable. He is very much in need of an intensive, well-coordinated program aimed at increasing his capacity for dealing with all aspects of behavioral control. Alterations in requirements for graphomotor output and efforts to desensitize him to the use of a pencil would appear to be in order. Concomitant efforts to deal with his very apparent socioemotional difficulties are essential. In all of this, it should be emphasized that this boy has a number of well-developed and even superior adaptive skills and abilities, which should be of considerable assistance in his attempts to adapt to remedial programming.

Postscript

John was admitted to a program that specializes in day treatment of children with LD and significant psychosocial difficulties. As mentioned above, his response to this program has been quite positive.

The recommendations that flowed from his neuropsychological assessment were seen as helpful in choosing appropriate therapeutic modalities/programs (e.g., Think Aloud) for him.

CASE 2: ANDREW

Relevance

At the time of referral for neuropsychological assessment, this 9-year, 7-month-old youngster was doing poorly in school. The neuropsychological assessment determined that Andrew does not have any type of LD, at least as we typically define such. He does have considerable difficulty in maintaining attention for even fairly brief periods of time, and he exhibits a significant degree of psychosocial dysfunction of the externalized variety.

In this case, we see poor school performance that appears to be caused by a combination of a disorder in attention deployment and a significant degree of socioemotional disturbance. As such, the relationships that obtain vis-à-vis Andrew's learning problems are of the sort characterized by Hypothesis 1 explanations.

Again, we present the results of the neuropsychological assessment in quasi-report format.

Neuropsychological Assessment Findings

Behavioral Observations during the Examination

Throughout the day-long testing session, Andrew was friendly with the examiner, and rapport was easily obtained and maintained with him. For the most part, he was attentive to the tasks at hand; however, there were many occasions when he did not focus his attention well. At times, he exhibited a somewhat below-average amount of verbal interchange with the examiner; at other times, he was quite verbose. There were occasions when he required considerable encouragement from the examiner to proceed with the tasks at hand. There were several occasions when he exhibited a rather low level of tolerance for frustration. He sometimes resisted providing guesses for questions about which he was unsure. His general level and quality of motor coordination were normal; there was a more than ordinary degree of irrelevant physical activity in evidence. His motivation to do well on the tests administered to him was, for the most part, adequate. However, there were many occasions when he refused to continue with tasks that he found difficult. It was also apparent that he was often quite resistant to the examiner's instructions. There were instances where he perseverated in erroneous responses, despite the examiner's urgings to modify his approach to the task at hand.

All things considered, it would appear that a fairly reliable estimate of this boy's adaptive skills and abilities was obtained in this examination. However, it is apparent that lower-bound estimates of his skills and abilities were probably elicited in some areas when his attentional deployment and/or cooperation with the instructions of the examiner were less than optimal.

Summary of Test Results and Impressions

General Comments. Andrew exhibited a wide range of well-developed skills and abilities. Those deficits that were in evidence were not consistent, and would not be compatible with any pattern of performance that is usually seen in children of this age who are suffering from central processing deficiencies. The deficits in evidence would appear to be explicable in terms of attention deployment difficulties and, more important, problems in complying with the examiner's instructions and the demands of the tasks before him. This situation is further complicated by his apparent difficulties in socioemotional functioning, primarily of the externalized variety. The following report was designed to add some specifications to these generalizations and to suggest some avenues to pursue in remedial programming for him. Figure 5.2 provides a summary of Andrew's test results.

Test Results and Impressions. There were no indications of any simple tactile imperception or suppression with either hand. Andrew experienced much more than ordinary difficulties in identifying symbols written on the fingertips of both hands. It would seem quite probable that problems in attention deployment and motivation posed the greatest difficulties for him on this task. There was no evidence of finger agnosia. He exhibited some difficulties in identifying coins placed within the right hand.

On a nonverbal problem-solving task (Tactual Performance Test, involving strategy generation, psychomotor coordination, and the capacity to benefit from tactile input and kinesthetic feedback), Andrew's level of performance with the left hand was mildly impaired; that with the right hand was within normal limits. His level of performance on a third trial of this task (using both hands together) was superior. His incidental memory for the shapes of the blocks used on this task was outstanding; however, he experienced difficulty in locating them properly on a drawing of the formboard. The very irregular pattern of performance evident on this task would suggest strongly that factors other than information-processing deficiencies were responsible for his isolated poor levels of performance on it.

Andrew would appear to be predominantly left-handed and exclusively left-footed and left-eyed. Strength of grip with the left hand was average; that with the right hand was well above average. A similar pattern of performance was evident on a test for finger-tapping speed with each hand. He performed approximately within normal limits on a test for foot-tapping speed. He performed extremely well on a test specifically designed for the measurement of static tremor. He did not comply with instructions for performance on a test designed for the measurement of kinetic tremor. Speeded eye–hand coordination on the Grooved Pegboard Test was average with the right hand and well below average with the left hand. Once again, the very irregular pattern of performance on this task would suggest strongly that factors other than information-processing deficiencies were responsible for Andrew's isolated poor levels of performance on it.

There were no indications of any simple visual imperception or suppression. He performed at a mildly impaired level on a test requiring immediate memory for visual sequences (Target Test); it would appear quite probable that lapses in attention deployment interfered with his performance on this test.

Andrew's graphic renderings of simple visual designs were marginally adequate from a visual–spatial perspective: All were

FIGURE 5.2. Summary of neuropsychological test results for Case 2 (Andrew).

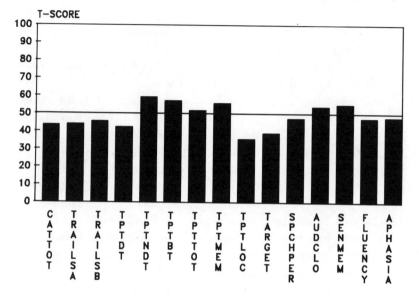

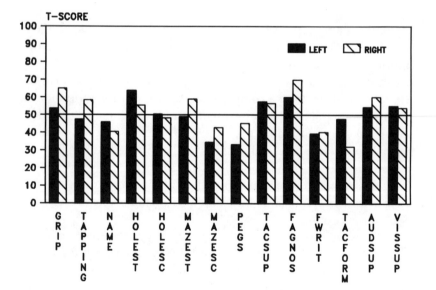

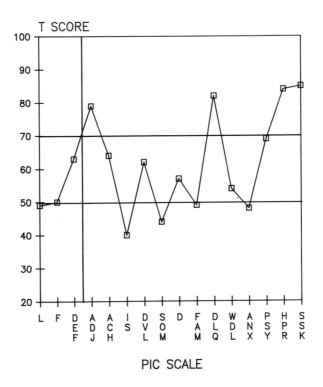

PIC SCALE

Test	Score at 9 yr, 7 mo
WISC-R	
Verbal IQ	106
Information	12
Comprehension	8
Arithmetic	10
Similarities	12
Vocabulary	13
Digit Span	9
Performance IQ	98
Picture Completion	11
Picture Arrangement	11
Block Design	13
Object Assembly	10
Coding	4
Full Scale IQ	102
PPVT IQ	112
WRAT-R	
Reading	91
Spelling	94
Arithmetic	91

marked by some evidence of tremor. Although rather neat in appearance, and approached and carried out with great care, his cursive script was also marked by some tremor. His drawing of a complex key was quite immature and lacking in visual–spatial detail; there were also some distortions of detail in evidence. It is probable that his difficulties in graphomotor skills relate to problems in complying with task demands and a degree of resistance that is quite out of the ordinary for children of his age.

On a task that required the use of a pencil and the rendering of fine visual discriminations under timed conditions (Underlining Test), he experienced considerable difficulty on some subtests, and performed quite well on others. It is probable that the requirement for speeded performance (which he generally resisted forcefully throughout this examination), especially when using a pencil, was the element of this task that posed considerable difficulties for him.

On the Performance section of the WISC-R, Andrew obtained a PIQ of 98. Subtest scaled scores on this section of the WISC-R ranged from a low of 4 on the Coding subtest to a high of 13 on the Block Design subtest. As was the case for other tests in this battery, the speeded requirement of the Coding subtest (wherein a pencil is used) was resisted by him. It is quite probable that Andrew does not have any information-processing deficiencies within the visual–spatial–organizational realm.

Andrew experienced some mild difficulties on a task (Trail Making Test) that required him to negotiate a visual–spatial array with a pencil on the basis of the numeric sequence. When this test was rendered somewhat more complex by the addition of the requirement to alternate between the numeric and alphabetic sequences in order to complete the task, his level of performance was normal.

There were no indications of any simple auditory imperception or suppression with either ear. Performance on a Sweep Hearing Test was within normal limits. He experienced somewhat more than ordinary difficulty on a task requiring fine auditory discrimination and sustained attentional skills (Seashore Rhythm Test). It is probable that he did not comply completely with the task demands of this test.

Andrew performed within normal limits on a test for sound blending. He experienced no difficulty on a test for verbatim memory for sentences; in this particular instance, the requirement for sustained attention to the sentences posed no difficulties for him. He exhibited normal levels of performance on a phonemically cued test of verbal fluency and on a test that required him to underline the graphic equivalents of novel speech sounds.

On the PPVT, Andrew obtained a Mental Age of 11 years, 4 months, which is equivalent to an IQ of 112.

On the Verbal section of the WISC-R, Andrew obtained a VIQ of 106. Subtest scaled scores on this section of the WISC-R ranged from lows of 8 on the Comprehension subtest and 9 on the Digit Span subtest to a high of 13 on the Vocabulary subtest. This particular pattern of subtest scaled scores, in conjunction with his other average levels of performance on verbal and language-related tasks, would suggest strongly that Andrew's basic psycholinguistic capacities are developed to a normal degree for his age.

Andrew exhibited no clear indications of any aphasic deficits on the Aphasia Screening Test. He did exhibit more than ordinary difficulties with the spelling of age-appropriate words. There was a naming error in evidence, but this is very difficult to explain in view of his quite normal levels of performance on any number of verbal tasks; also, it was an isolated instance of naming difficulties.

On a very complex nonverbal problem-solving task (Category Test, involving concept formation, strategy generation, and the capacity to benefit from positive and negative informational feedback), his level of performance was somewhat poor. His noncompliance with the instructions for this task (which were repeated by the examiner several times) would appear to account for this poor level of performance.

On the WRAT-R, Andrew obtained the following approximate grade-equivalent (centile) scores: Reading, 3 (27); Spelling, 3 (34); Arithmetic, 3 (27). Most of his misspellings were of the phonetically accurate variety. On the Reading subtest, his approach to the decoding of words was largely of the "sight-word/best-guess" variety (e.g., "quietly" for "quality," "shook" for "struck," "carefully" for "clarify"). His performance on the Arithmetic subtest suggests that he has mastered some of the elementary principles relating to the basic arithmetic calculation skills of addition, subtraction, and multiplication. However, his performance was somewhat inconsistent on this subtest.

On the PIC (completed by his mother), there were some indications that Andrew is perceived as suffering from some degree of socioemotional disturbance (perhaps predominantly of the acting-out or externalized variety). Similarly, there were clear indications on an activity rating scale and on a behavior problem checklist that he is perceived as exhibiting a number of behavior problems of the latter variety, together with some that would be characterized as internalized forms of psychopathology. It is notable that the mother's responses on the PIC did not suggest that she is especially concerned about Andrew's difficulties within the academic realm.

Neuropsychological Disposition and Implications

This particular pattern of neuropsychological test results would not tend to raise any particular question regarding the functional integrity of Andrew's brain. The clinical picture is one that is compatible with the operation of patterns of resistance and other socioemotional difficulties that have become habitual for this boy. It is probable that his periodic problems in attention deployment are a reflection of problems within the socioemotional realm.

Andrew would be expected to experience considerable difficulty in attempting to learn within a normal or standard academic environment. He is very much in need of some form of psychotherapeutic/behavioral intervention if he is to make satisfactory progress in any realm of adaptive functioning. (At this point we did not have enough information to suggest whether or not Andrew's mother was also in need of some assistance along these lines.)

Postscript

Andrew was seen as in need of the type of behavioral interventions that are discussed at length by Barkley (1981). These were applied. In addition, Andrew's mother was trained in the use of the "directive parental counseling" method designed by Holland (1983). This combination of treatments was reasonably effective in dealing with Andrew's problems in attention deployment within the academic realm. Indeed, his academic performance improved rather dramatically within a few weeks of the application of these procedures. That some of his psychosocial difficulties (and, as it turned out, those of his mother) were related to issues that extended well beyond his apparently easily remediable academic difficulties necessitated the use of other, essentially "psychotherapeutic," forms of intervention. These interventions were directed principally to the psychosocial difficulties being experienced by his mother.

CASE 3: CHRIS

Relevance

This 9-year, 10-month-old youngster was referred for neuropsychological assessment because of outstanding difficulties in academic performance. Difficulties in some aspects of socioemotional functioning were also noted. In this particular case, aspects of auditory-verbal processing were found to be quite deficient. Indeed, the language-based form of LD that Chris was found to exhibit is most similar to the "basic phonological processing disorder" described by Rourke (1989, Ch. 8). Furthermore, the subtype of LD that Chris exhibits would appear to lie at the root of his academic performance problems: That is, his difficulties in reading, spelling, and arithmetic would appear to be directly attributable to his problems in information processing. The manner in which his information-processing problems map onto his psychosocial difficulties is somewhat more indirect and is described in the "Postscript" section of this case presentation.

Once again, we present the results of the neuropsychological assessment in a quasi-report format.

Neuropsychological Assessment Findings

Behavioral Observations during the Examination

Throughout the day-long testing session, Chris was cooperative and friendly with the examiner. However, several aspects of his response style tended to interfere with his performances. Principal among these was the very impulsive manner in which he answered most questions and his rather unreflective approach to many tasks. His motivation to do well on the tests administered was, for the most part, not in any doubt. However, he was somewhat careless in his approach to tasks on occasion. He exhibited average levels of general physical activity and psychomotor coordination. Although easily distracted, he was usually able to maintain attention when closely supervised. There were some occasions when he required encouragement to continue with tasks that he found difficult.

All things considered, it would appear that a fairly reliable estimate of this boy's adaptive skills and abilities was obtained in this examination. However, it is clear that his impulsive, unreflective response style led him to make errors on a number of occasions, and that his best possible performances may not have been obtained in such situations.

Summary of Test Results and Impressions

General Comments. Chris exhibited a number of difficulties in dealing with many aspects of psycholinguistic skill development. In addition to his impulsive response style, these difficulties would appear to be at the root of his problems in academic learning. He exhibited many well-developed skills and abilities, mostly of a non-verbal nature. There were no indications of any marked behavioral or socioemotional disturbances in evidence. It would appear that he is in need of specialized assistance if he is to make adequate progress in the academic setting. The following aspects of this report were designed to add some specifications to these generalizations. Figure 5.3 provides a summary of Chris's test results.

Test Results and Impressions. There were no indications of any simple tactile imperception or suppression with either hand. There were no problems in evidence on a test for finger localization. Chris experienced no particular difficulties in identifying coins by touch with either hand. He exhibited no more than ordinary difficulties in identifying numbers written on the fingertips of the each hand.

On a complex nonverbal problem-solving task (Tactual Performance Test, involving psychomotor coordination and the capacity to benefit from tactile input and kinesthetic feedback), this boy's overall level of performance was quite good. Chris gave every indication of being able to benefit from experience with this task. His incidental memory for the shapes of the blocks used on this task and for their proper locations on a drawing of the formboard was within normal limits. It is clear that this type of "hands-on" task, which restrains one sensory modality—in this case, the visual (by means of a blindfold)—constitutes one ideal learning environment for Chris.

There were no indications of any simple visual imperception or suppression. He performed very well on a task designed for the measurement of immediate memory for visual sequences (Target Test).

On the Performance section of the WISC-R, Chris obtained a PIQ of 106. Subtest scaled scores on this section of the WISC-R ranged from lows of 10 on the Picture Arrangement and Coding subtests to a high of 13 on the Picture Completion subtest. It is clear that the visual–spatial–organizational skills and abilities that this section of the WISC-R was designed to measure are normally developed.

On the Underlining Test (a measure that requires rapid information processing for a variety of verbal and nonverbal target items), his overall level of performance was mildly impaired. Chris experienced particular difficulty when he was required to deal with verbal target items; nonverbal target stimuli posed no serious problems for him on this test. It is apparent that Chris experienced difficulty in dealing with the symbolic aspects of stimuli that must be perceived and processed under timed conditions.

On a task that required him to negotiate a visual–spatial array on the basis of alternations between the numeric and alphabetic sequences (Trail Making Test), he performed within normal limits.

Chris would appear to be predominantly right-handed, right-footed, and left-eyed. Strength of grip was average with the right and left hands. Simple motor speed was well above normal limits with both hands. Foot-tapping speeds were somewhat poor. There was some evidence of static tremor, especially with the left hand. His performances with both hands on tasks specifically designed for the measurement of kinetic tremor were within normal limits. Speeded eye–hand coordination (as measured with the Grooved Pegboard Test) with both hands was within normal limits, and in the expected relationship for a right-handed individual.

FIGURE 5.3. Summary of neuropsychological test results for Case 3 (Chris).

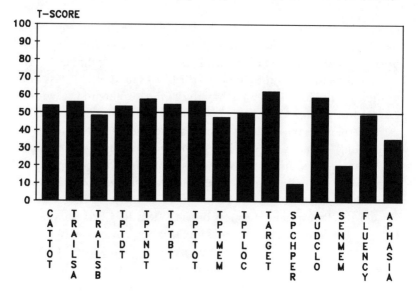

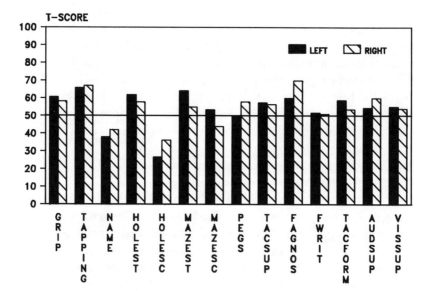

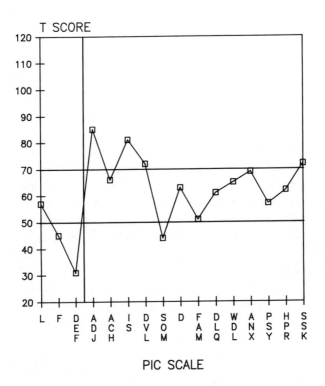

T SCORE

PIC SCALE

Test	Score at 9 yr, 10 mo
WISC-R	
Verbal IQ	84
Information	7
Comprehension	8
Arithmetic	7
Similarities	8
Vocabulary	7
Digit Span	6
Performance IQ	106
Picture Completion	13
Picture Arrangement	10
Block Design	11
Object Assembly	11
Coding	10
Full Scale IQ	93
PPVT IQ	84
WRAT-R	
Reading	74
Spelling	69
Arithmetic	86

His printing and his cursive script were both rather immature and marked by a very mild degree of tremor. Tremor was also evident in his graphic reproductions of simple visual designs. There were no clear-cut visual–spatial distortions evident in his renderings of these designs. However, Chris had difficulty in reproducing the intricate details in a drawing of a key; this is often seen in children of this age who experience problems in directing their behavior by verbal means.

There were no indications of any simple auditory imperception or suppression. A Sweep Hearing Test did not reveal any indications of deficiencies in auditory acuity. He performed somewhat below normal limits on a task requiring fine auditory discrimination and sustained attentional capacities (Seashore Rhythm Test).

On a test designed for the measurement of sound blending, Chris performed within normal limits. Phonemically cued verbal fluency was average. He experienced considerable difficulty on a test requiring verbatim memory for sentences of gradually increasing length; problems with distractibility may very well have compromised his performance on this test. His level of performance on a task requiring him to underline the graphic equivalents of novel speech sounds was severely impaired.

He obtained a VIQ of 84 on the Verbal section of the WISC-R. Subtest scaled scores on this section of the WISC-R ranged from a low of 6 on the Digit Span subtest to highs of 8 on the Comprehension and Similarities subtests. This particular pattern of subtest scaled scores is often seen in children of this age who are experiencing difficulties in psycholinguistic skill development that are hampering their attempts at learning basic academic subjects. Difficulties in dealing with short bursts of nonredundant verbal information are often characteristic of such youngsters, as are problems in dealing adaptively with the phonological structure of spoken and written words.

On the Aphasia Screening Test, Chris exhibited clear difficulties in spelling and reading age-appropriate words and in the enunciation of complex multisyllabic words. There were also some indications of difficulties in simple arithmetic calculation. There were no naming errors in evidence. There were some indications of auditory–verbal agnosia.

Chris obtained a Mental Age of 7 years, 10 months (equivalent to an IQ of 84) on the PPVT.

On the WRAT-R, he obtained the following approximate

grade-equivalent (centile) scores: Reading, 2 (4); Spelling, 2 (2); Arithmetic, 3 (18). Most of his misspellings were of the phonetically accurate variety. Virtually all of his reading errors were of the "sight-word/best-guess" variety (e.g., "lamp" for "lame," "chief" for "cliff," "quickly" for "quality"). It is clear that Chris experiences considerable difficulty in using a phonetic word attack strategy for the reading of unfamiliar words. Also, his impulsive response style may very well hamper him in the utilization of such a systematic, labored approach to word decoding. His performance on the Arithmetic subtest was at a level somewhat below that which would be expected on the basis of his performances on tests involving the components of arithmetic calculation abilities. Problems in (verbal) memory for arithmetic procedures and in reading the arithmetic questions would appear to have played a significant role in his difficulties on this subtest.

On a very complex nonverbal problem-solving task (Category Test, involving concept formation, hypothesis testing, and the capacity to benefit from positive and negative informational feedback), his overall level of performance approached the upper limits of the normal range. It is clear that he was well able to utilize the (nonverbal) corrective informational feedback available in this test, in spite of his tendency to respond quickly and without much reflection.

His mother's responses on rating scales for hyperactivity and common behavior problems suggest that she does not perceive Chris as overly active in most situations or susceptible to any significant form or degree of socioemotional difficulties. Her responses on the PIC were not suggestive of any significant degree of perceived psychopathology. However, the mother did express some concerns regarding her son's capacity to follow often-repeated instructions, his apparent unwillingness to accept responsibility for untoward actions, and his problems in making and keeping friends.

Neuropsychological Disposition and Implications

Although clearly not diagnostic of any neuropathological disease process, this particular pattern of neuropsychological test results would be compatible with long-term, chronic dysfunction at the level of the cerebral hemispheres. There were no indications in this profile of neuropsychological test results that would be compatible with the presence of any acute neurological disease process. Abilities and skills ordinarily thought to be subserved primarily by the temporal–parietal region of the left cerebral hemisphere would appear to be particularly compromised.

Chris experiences much difficulty in a variety of situations that require him to attend to and assimilate short bursts of nonredundant auditory–verbal information. This sort of demand comes to characterize the academic situation more and more with advancing years. Since he requires much in the way of multimodal, redundant instruction, with an abundance of corrective feedback in order to make progress in learning, it would appear probable that placement within a "regular" academic milieu would not meet his information-processing needs. Indeed, it would be expected that Chris would fall further and further behind with respect to academic learning in such a setting. Feelings of self-worth and other important socioemotional dimensions of behavior may suffer if his specific information-processing needs are not met in the academic milieu. Although there is no evidence to suggest that any untoward psychosocial difficulties are *necessary* consequences of Chris's particular form of LD, it would be well to note that the emotional strain associated with prolonged failure can interact with a less than satisfactory family and school support system to increase the probability of such an occurrence.

It is apparent that Chris has many well-developed skills and abilities, particularly within the nonverbal realm. It is important that the development of these skills and abilities be encouraged, and that he come to realize that accomplishments within these areas are valued by those whose opinion he respects. Within the academic milieu, it would seem advisable to encourage such development by accentuating his average to above-average skills and abilities in the projects that are assigned to him.

Postscript

It may well be instructive to give an example of the manner in which this youngster's information processing and psychosocial functioning interact. We do so within the context of explaining briefly how we dealt with what Chris's mother mentioned as a problem that caused her a considerable amount of difficulty— namely, his "disobedience."

His mother had long thought that Chris might be "deaf." When she spoke to him from another room, or from behind him, or when any degree of ambient noise was present, it was as if he did not hear her: Chris simply went about his business with no regard to what she had said. His mother was made aware of this, and she promptly changed her instruction-giving behavior to the manner that was suggested to her. This involved the following: (1) delivering instructions only after she was standing in front of him and had gained his undivided attention; (2) delivering instructions in simple, straightforward prose; and (3) asking him to repeat or paraphrase instructions before proceeding with the behaviors that he had been asked to perform. We emphasized that instructions should be kept short and to the point, and should be accompanied by suitable facial expressions and other appropriate nonverbal gesticulations. Furthermore, we emphasized that no performance should be initiated by Chris until he described accurately what he was expected to do.

The mother was surprised to learn that such procedures were very effective. She found that his previous "bull-headedness" all but disappeared. And she was encouraged to view this as a fairly simple process: Once Chris understood and was able to verbalize what was expected of him, he was quite prepared and able to undertake the instruction in question.

CASE 4: JANE

Relevance

This case report covers five neuropsychological examinations of a girl who exhibits the syndrome of nonverbal learning disabilities (NLD). Jane's test results are presented for the following reasons: (1) They represent a good example of the "developmental presentation" of this subtype of LD—that is, the one most likely to be encountered by the practicing clinician; (2) the changes in the presentation of the NLD syndrome over the approximately 8 years of follow-up that the test results represent are of interest; (3) the interaction between Jane's neuropsychological assets and deficits on the one hand, and her patterns of academic achievement and psychosocial functioning on the other, is illustrated; and (4) the possible impact of intensive treatment on the presentation of the NLD syndrome is discernible. In all of this, we attempt to emphasize that Jane's NLD lie at the root of all of her adaptive problems, including those within the psychosocial realm.

Relevant History

Jane was referred for neuropsychological assessment by her family physician. She was said to be experiencing problems in communicating through writing, and her mechanical arithmetic skills were reported to be very weak. In addition, it was reported that her fine and gross motor abilities were very poorly developed. On the other hand, her oral reading and spelling abilities were described as quite good. At the time of the initial assessment, she was 9 years, 6 months of age, and she was enroled in a regular grade 4 program. Her mother reported that Jane had difficulties with concentration, and she also expressed concern regarding Jane's ability to relate to other children.

Inspection of Jane's history revealed that she was the first-born child, delivered after a full-term pregnancy by caesarian section. A trial of labor had been carried out prior to this procedure. Jane was nursed for 24 hours in an incubator and later on in a normal crib. For the most part, her course through infancy was unremarkable, although at 14 months of age it was noted that her motor coordination and vocabulary were somewhat delayed. She had no serious illnesses during infancy and childhood, except for a few febrile episodes, during one or two of which she became somewhat delirious. She was also under medical care for possible allergies.

Neuropsychological Assessment Findings

Jane underwent comprehensive neuropsychological evaluations on four occasions: at the ages of 9 years, 6 months; 11 years, 0 months;

12 years, 11 months; and 15 years, 5 months. She was also examined on a more circumscribed basis at the age of 17 years, 8 months. The data for the first four comprehensive neuropsychological examinations are contained in Figure 5.4. Of particular importance in this presentation are the stability of Jane's neuropsychological status over time, the evidence of her positive response to a program of therapy/intervention, and her residual difficulties in adaptive functioning at the age of almost 18 years.

Behavioral Observations during the Examinations

During the initial, day-long assessment (at 9 years, 6 months), Jane was reasonably cooperative and friendly with the examiner; rapport was easily established with her. However, she seemed to be somewhat distractible, exhibiting difficulties with attention deployment. She often required guidance and encouragement in order to exert her best efforts; the exception to this was her rather enthusiastic approach to tasks of a clearly verbal (academic-like) nature. She required considerable instruction, assistance, and practice in order to complete motoric and visual–spatial tasks as required. She was quite loquacious; however, her conversation was rather inappropriate, tangential, and often unrelated to the task at hand. Her gait was awkward, and her general level of motor coordination was noticeably poor. It should be clear from this description of her ambient behavior during this examination that she exhibited many characteristics that we have come to associate with children who exhibit the NLD syndrome (see Chapter 4, this volume, and Rourke, 1989).

Throughout the second examination, at the age of 11 years, 0 months, Jane was reasonably friendly, talkative, and cooperative; rapport was easily obtained with her. However, there was some evidence of slight distractibility and carelessness, and on some occasions she seemed to give up on tasks that she perceived as too difficult. It was fairly obvious from her performance on paper-and-pencil tasks that her eye–hand coordination was quite poor. She seemed to have particular difficulty in starting lines on the left side of the page, apparently because she experienced problems in controlling her hand movement from the end of one line (on the right side) to the beginning of the next line (on the left side). Another

FIGURE 5.4. Summary of neuropsychological test results for Case 4 (Jane).

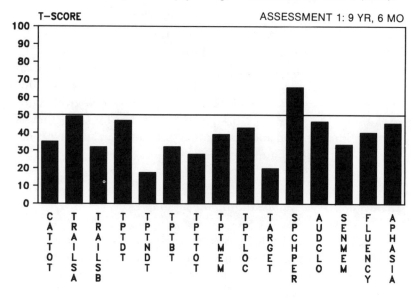

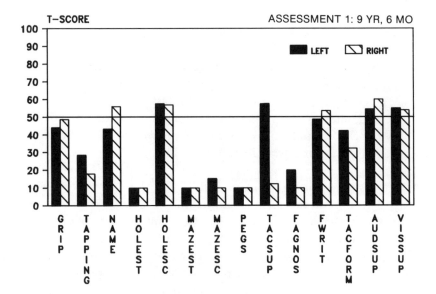

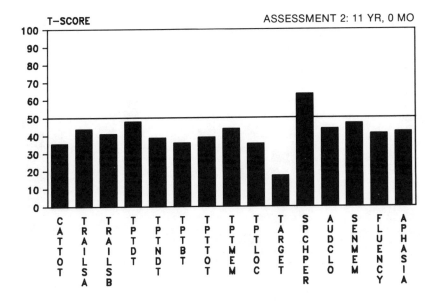

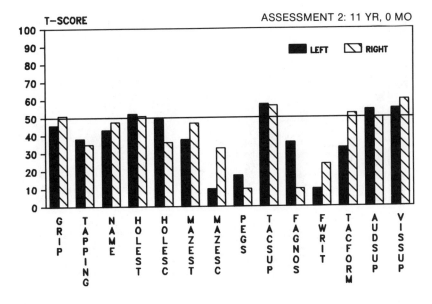

(continued)

FIGURE 5.4. (continued)

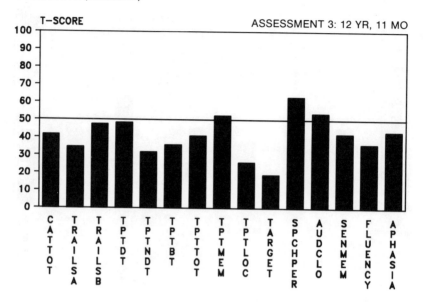

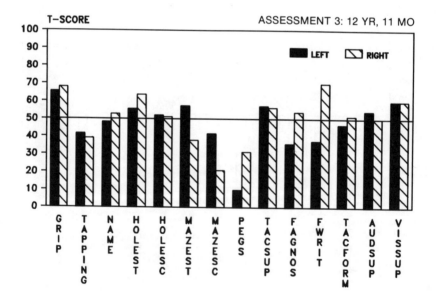

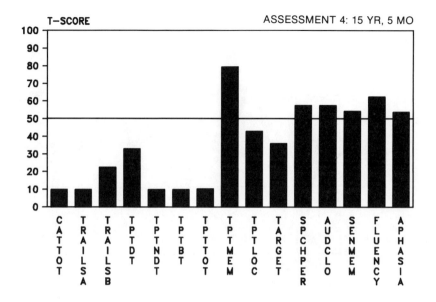

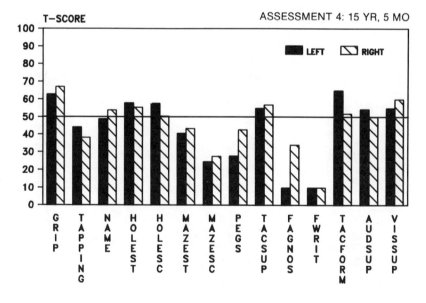

(continued)

FIGURE 5.4. (continued)

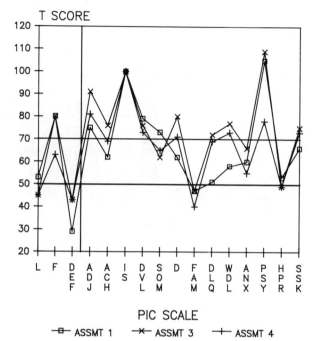

PIC SCALE

Test	Score at:			
	9 yr, 6 mo	11 yr, 0 mo	12 yr, 11 mo	15 yr, 5 mo
WISC				
Verbal IQ	101	97	105	101
Information	9	11	10	8
Comprehension	8	6	7	10
Arithmetic	8	6	8	7
Similarities	11	13	13	11
Vocabulary	13	10	10	8
Digit Span	12	12	17	17
Performance IQ	75	80	86	79
Picture Completion	8	6	8	7
Picture Arrangement	8	9	12	9
Block Design	6	9	9	8
Object Assembly	6	8	6	6
Coding	4	4	5	5
Full Scale IQ	88	88	96	90
PPVT IQ	99	113	112	na
WRAT				
Reading	141	141	107	115
Spelling	116	131	110	109
Arithmetic	85	89	71	78

notable feature of her behavior in this second examination was a rather different, "sing-song" quality to her voice.

In the fourth examination, at the age of 15 years, 5 months, Jane was very cooperative and very talkative. Her motivation to do well on the tests administered was never in any doubt. In general, she was somewhat hypoactive. Occasionally, she became somewhat distracted from the task at hand; this took the form of "drifting off" during passive attending conditions. At such times, she seemed to be unaware that stimuli were being presented to her. It is notable that this distractibility was confined almost exclusively to those situations involving the presentation of visual stimuli. Her general level of motor coordination, especially when walking or engaged in fine manipulatory activities, was quite poor. On several occasions she exhibited rather immature behavior, although her general approach to the testing situation was one of compliance and cooperation. It is clear that her ambient behavior at the time of this fourth testing was quite typical of that seen in children who exhibit the NLD syndrome (Rourke, 1989).

Neurological Examination Results at 10 Years

Electroencephalographic (EEG) evaluation was not particularly helpful in this case. The tracing obtained was judged to be essentially within normal limits, except for some nonspecific, generalized mild dysrhythmia emanating from both cerebral hemispheres. Activation did not provoke any focal abnormality or epileptic activity. Physical neurological examination revealed mild ataxia and apraxia, with the latter appearing to be more marked on the left side. Jane also exhibited a marked nystagmus on gaze to the left. Otherwise, the neurological examination was unremarkable. On the basis of these findings, a neurologist suggested possible mild cerebellar–pontine dysfunction. A question was also raised regarding possible endocrine dysfunction because of the generalized distribution of adipose tissue.

Treatment/Intervention Program

Following her first neuropsychological assessment, Jane entered a day treatment program on a full-time basis. She spent 5 years in this program. Following this experience, she was enroled in a residential treatment program for approximately 2 years. In both programs, there was a heavy emphasis on life skills training, psychomotor development, counseling, and appropriate-level academic training. Especially during the initial 5-year day treatment placement, these efforts were guided by the principles and procedures outlined more extensively elsewhere (Rourke, 1989; Strang & Rourke, 1985a). It is important to emphasize the intensive nature of the treatment programs in which Jane was involved over the 7-year period in question when interpreting the neuropsychological assessment results available during this time frame.

Assessment Results and Clinical Observations

In her first comprehensive neuropsychological examination at 9 years, 6 months of age (see Figure 5.4), it was quite clear that Jane exhibited the major neuropsychological, academic, and socioemotional features of the NLD syndrome. Indeed, there were few deviations from this pattern in evidence. In view of this, a treatment/ intervention program was commenced. This program, as noted above, took the form of full-time day treatment in a center specializing in the care of learning-disabled children who have associated mental health needs.

The results of the second examination (at 11 years, 0 months) indicated that Jane had made considerable gains in a number of areas of adaptive functioning. The most notable of these were in the areas of motor steadiness, motor coordination, problem-solving attack strategies, spelling, and some elements of attention deployment. However, it was equally clear that she continued to experience rather marked visual–spatial and visual–organizational difficulties, together with problems in short-term memory for visual sequences. Although her drawings of geometric forms remained slightly distorted, there were indications of some improvement in her capacity to organize visual–spatial output. Although eye–hand coordination had improved somewhat, it remained enough of a problem for her that her performance under speeded conditions continued to be an area of concern. As was observed in the first assessment, Jane exhibited rather well-developed skills in reading (word recognition) and spelling, but mechanical arithmetic remained an area of relative academic weakness. She was able to add, subtract, and multiply in a competent manner, but division still posed difficulty for her.

As a result of this second assessment, it was felt that a continuation of her therapeutic program was in order. There was every indication that the specific training that commenced at the conclusion of the first assessment seemed to have helped her in many areas of adaptive functioning; at the very least, there were no compelling indications of deterioration in her most deficient areas of adaptive functioning.

Aside from her obvious academic difficulties, especially in the area of arithmetic, a major problem faced by Jane involved her poorly developed social skills. Indeed, at the age of 12 years, 11 months, she obtained a social age equivalent to 8 years, 3 months, and a social quotient of 69 on the Vineland Social Maturity Scale (Doll, 1953). Personnel at the treatment center in which she was enroled described her as being friendly with adults and tending to seek their praise and acknowledgment in an active manner. However, they also reported that she responded to social interactions in a rather automatic fashion, with only a limited expression of meaningful affect. Her relationships with peers were certainly less than ideal. Peer interactions were often characterized by silly, inappropriate verbalizations on her part.

It is clear that the major factor in Jane's poorly developed social skills related to her inability to interpret appropriate nonverbal sources of communication (such as facial expressions, body postures, and various gestures). She would be expected to be at considerable risk for misinterpreting or failing to interpret many relevant elements in social situations.

Despite the difficulties that Jane exhibited at 11 and 12 years of age, it was also clear that the intensive treatment program provided for her had paid some dividends. Test–retest comparisons indicated dramatic improvements in her motor and psychomotor skills. In addition, it was quite clear that her capacity to attend to auditory stimulation had increased, although this did not appear to be the case within the visual–spatial or tactile–perceptual realms. Visual scanning and tracking remained a problem; while this did not appear to affect the reading of single words, it may have interfered with her capacity to extract meaning from reading passages. It was evident that Jane was very adept at associating and defining words, although the associations that she made to words often tended to be rather bizarre.

Prior to treatment, she had very few positive socializing experiences outside of her immediate family unit. Her experience in the treatment program, in addition to providing an opportunity to develop her academic skills, undoubtedly contributed to a more positive social experience for her. Because of the many positive gains that Jane exhibited as a result of treatment, plans were formulated to find a placement for her in a regular school system. Unfortunately, this did not turn out to be a clinically viable tack to follow. Indeed, reports from her parents and her caretakers in the treatment program continued to indicate that she was not "ready" to take this step. Trials of partial integration within the regular school system were orchestrated carefully and with considerable cooperation from the school in question. However, repeated observations by all of those involved in her care led to the conclusion that Jane would need the support of a treatment center and program for the foreseeable future.

In order to cast some light on why this turned out to be the case, it is instructive to consider the results of her fourth neuropsychological assessment, at the age of 15 years, 5 months. These are best described in terms of a set of comparisons with the results obtained in her first assessment, as follows:

1. In general, the results of the first and fourth examinations were quite similar. This was especially apparent in the areas of Jane's principal neuropsychological deficiencies (e.g., as measured with the Performance subtests of the WISC and with the Category Test [adult version administered in the fourth examination]).

2. It should be noted that there were some changes in a positive direction in some of her expected areas of neuropsychological strength, such as simple motor skills (e.g., grip strength, finger-tapping speed), rote verbal skills (e.g., WISC Digit Span, Auditory Closure Test), and other verbal receptive skills (e.g., the PPVT).

3. Her improved performance on the Tactual Performance Test suggested that her therapy/intervention program may have been most helpful in those skill and ability areas that are important for the successful completion of this task, especially the ability to utilize

tactile-kinesthetic information to guide her motor performance. However, despite these gains, note should be taken of the persistence since the first assessment of the pattern of relative performance deficiency with the left hand.

4. The persistence of Jane's patterns of performance over time is quite remarkable, especially when one considers that this occurred in the academic areas (high reading and spelling, low arithmetic), the "verbal" versus visual–spatial–organizational areas, and patterns of socioemotional responsivity.

5. However, with respect to the latter, it should be noted that Jane's PIC results do reflect some encouraging gains (see especially the much lower elevation on the Psychosis scale).

Jane's clinical picture at the time of the fourth assessment contained a number of rather significant and encouraging positive developments, which presumably were a function of the rather intensive therapy/intervention program in which she had been participating. However, the Vineland Adaptive Behavior Scales (VABS; Sparrow, Balla, & Cicchetti, 1984) results at the time of her fifth testing (Table 5.1) were not reflective of a capacity for completely independent living at that time. These results are indeed somewhat discouraging, in that they point to a number of adaptive areas within which Jane made very little progress over time. More

TABLE 5.1. Vineland Adaptive Behavior Scales Results for Jane and Gerry

	Standard score	Centile	Age equivalent
Jane (17 yr, 8 mo)			
Communication	48	<1	8 yr, 10 mo
Daily Living	57	<1	8 yr, 10 mo
Socialization	47	<1	8 yr, 10 mo
Motor (estimates)			4 yr, 3 mo
Adaptive Behavior Composite	47	<1	7 yr, 3 mo
Maladaptive Behavior	Raw score = 13; significant		
Gerry (16 yr, 4 mo)			
Communication	70	2	10 yr, 10 mo
Daily Living	78	7	11 yr, 9 mo
Socialization	69	2	10 yr, 4 mo
Motor (estimates)			>5 yr, 11 mo
Adaptive Behavior Composite	67	1	11 yr, 0 mo
Maladaptive Behavior	Raw score = 13; significant		

generally, it is often the case that the VABS results of NLD youngsters are more pervasively and more significantly impaired than are
those of their brain-damaged age-mates who have sustained very
significant cerebral lesions that have not had a widespread negative
impact on white matter functioning.

In order to illustrate the latter point, the VABS results of a 16-
year-old youngster are also reported in Table 5.1. This boy (Gerry)
had sustained a very severe stroke involving the middle region of the
left cerebral hemisphere. The bleeding and subsequent necrosis of
tissue within this region left him with very severe aphasic sympto-
matology (similar to the disconnection syndrome) and marked motoric limitations on the right side of the body. In spite of these
deficiencies, his VABS scores were generally superior to those of
Jane. (For a more complete analysis of this particular case, see Ch. 2
of Rourke, Fisk, & Strang, 1986.)

Jane and Gerry: Social/Vocational Outcomes

It is also instructive to consider and compare the current social and
vocational status of Jane and Gerry. At this writing, at the age of
21 years, Jane is involved in a "career search" that is proceeding
reasonably well. She is receiving considerable support in this effort
from a number of individuals, including her parents. She is thought
to have achieved a marginal level of adjustment, but the earmarks of
the NLD syndrome (especially in the areas of judgment and reasoning) persist. It is clear that her limitations in these areas will continue to pose substantial limitations in her social and vocational
life. Gerry, at the age of 21, is still quite frankly aphasic. However,
he is seen as quite well adjusted and socially adaptive. One pursuit
in which he has been engaged has involved assisting handicapped
individuals in the use of computers as part of their therapy programs. Gerry is quite adept at this teaching enterprise, and is found
to be well liked by his "students." His own computer is pro-
grammed with a variety of software, which he can access on demand
when his word-finding skills fail him. He is quite adept at deciding
when he needs access to such material, and manages to do so
without alienating those around him. These few observations
should be sufficient to suggest that the modes of adaptation for Jane

and Gerry are quite different, and that the prognosis for social and vocational adjustment is significantly more positive for Gerry than for Jane.

Summary of Test Results and Implications

Jane's neuropsychological protocol is marked by a pattern of impaired visual–spatial skills, some tactile–perceptual difficulties, deficient problem-solving and concept formation abilities, impaired psychomotor functioning, and relatively intact rote verbal skills. The principal point to be made in this connection is that Jane's pattern of test results is quite typical of the "developmental" presentation of the NLD syndrome. In spite of her average to superior levels of performance in some areas, she is still facing significant social and vocational difficulties. Although it would appear to be the case that Jane's therapy/intervention program has been quite successful in a number of areas, it is clear that she still experiences very significant limitations in her adaptive capacities as an apparent reflection of the NLD syndrome.

In brief, this is a clear example of a "Hypothesis 3" situation: That is, Jane's academic and psychosocial functioning would appear to be a fairly direct reflection of the particular neuropsychological assets and deficits that constitute her particular subtype of LD. Furthermore, this case offers us the opportunity to examine and formulate hypotheses regarding the combined effects of (1) maturation, (2) interactions of her neuropsychological assets and deficits with the developmental demands of her environment, and (3) treatment. As mentioned on several occasions throughout this volume, we view this type of study as essential for determining the interrelationships that are the focus of the book.

CASE 5: CARLA

Relevance

This 6-year, 3-month-old girl presented with the early manifestations of the NLD syndrome. Virtually all of the characteristics associated with this syndrome were present. During the administration of the neuropsychological tests, Carla posed considerable challenges for the examiner, although sufficient data were obtained in order to arrive at some fairly clear conclusions regarding her adaptive difficulties and modes of intervention appropriate to address them. Shortly after this assessment, she entered a day treatment program that specializes in the care of children with LD and associated mental health disturbances. We have found that such a facility is ideal for the treatment of children with this subtype of LD, both with respect to academic/formal learning opportunities and with respect to the very salient psychosocial disabilities from which they suffer.

We return to a quasi-report format for the presentation of the neuropsychological data and formulations for this case. The format is somewhat different from that used in Cases 1, 2, and 3.

Neuropsychological Assessment Findings

Behavioral Observations during the Examination

Throughout the day-long testing session, Carla was somewhat uncooperative with the examiner, and consistent rapport was very difficult to obtain and maintain with her. She was frequently inattentive to the tasks at hand and exhibited some irrelevant physical activity. She exhibited an adequate amount of verbal interchange with the examiner; indeed, there were occasions when she talked a great deal. There was some evidence of enunciatory dyspraxia. There were many occasions when she required considerable encouragement to continue with the tasks at hand. Her general level of psychomotor coordination was very poor. Her motivation to do well on the tests administered was sometimes in doubt.

Summary of Test Results and Impressions

Reliability of the Test Results. In view of the difficulties evident throughout the testing sessions, it would appear highly probable that a completely reliable estimate of this girl's adaptive skills and abilities was not obtained. However, there were a number of patterns evident in her neuropsychological profile that allow for the generating of some confident assertions regarding her current levels of adaptive abilities and deficits.

General Observations. There were some general observations made throughout the testing sessions. Some of these are as follows: (1) Carla was able to identify almost all of the letters of the alphabet. (2) Paper-and-pencil tasks were quite poorly executed. In general, psychomotor tasks posed considerable difficulty for her. (3) There were several occasions when she became quite confused and unable to use even very simple strategies for solving problems. (4) Some of her verbalizations were very much off-topic. (5) There was clear evidence of a "warm-up" effect on a number of tasks. (6) Although her attention faltered often, she did not wander about or touch materials in the testing room; more generally, she did not appear to be at all interested in exploring the environment of the testing room. (7) Visual–spatial–organizational skills were very poorly developed. (8) Carla exhibited many very well-developed linguistic skills, mostly of a rote, overlearned nature.

A more detailed report of Carla's test results follows. These are also summarized in Figure 5.5.

Test-Specific Observations and General Conclusions. There were some borderline indications of simple tactile imperception with the left side of the face; there was also some evidence of tactile suppression with the right hand. Carla performed at mildly impaired to borderline levels on tests for finger agnosia and finger dysgraphesthesia. There was no evidence of astereognosis for forms with either hand.

On a complex nonverbal problem-solving task (Tactual Performance Test, involving psychomotor coordination and the capacity to benefit from tactile input and kinesthetic feedback), she was not able to make any progress. The elementary demands for strategy generation on this task appeared to pose considerable difficulty for her.

Carla would appear to be predominantly right-handed, left-footed, and left-eyed. Strength of grip with the upper extremities was average, and in the expected relationship for a right-handed

FIGURE 5.5. Summary of neuropsychological test results for Case 5 (Carla).

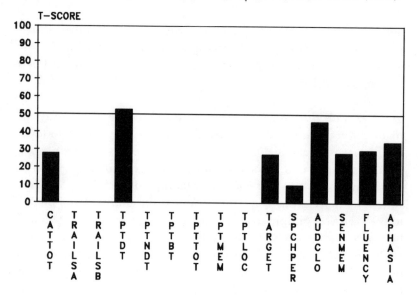

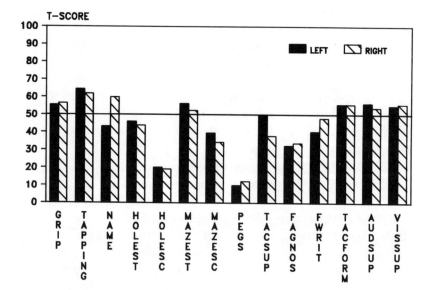

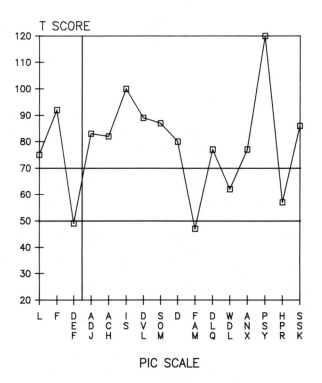

PIC SCALE

Test	Score at 6 yr, 3 mo
WISC-R	
Verbal IQ	94
Information	10
Comprehension	10
Arithmetic	6
Similarities	9
Vocabulary	10
Digit Span	1
Performance IQ	64
Picture Completion	4
Picture Arrangement	5
Block Design	6
Object Assembly	3
Coding	4
Full Scale IQ	77
PPVT IQ	111
WRAT-R	
Reading	89
Spelling	61
Arithmetic	80

child. Finger-tapping speed was above average with both hands. There was fairly clear evidence of static and kinetic tremor with both hands on tests specifically designed for the measurement of these dimensions. Speeded eye–hand coordination (Grooved Pegboard Test) was markedly impaired with both hands; this difficulty was somewhat more apparent with the left hand.

There were no clear indications of any simple visual imperception or suppression. She performed at a moderately impaired level on a test requiring immediate memory for visual sequences (Target Test).

Carla performed poorly on a task requiring her to match pictures on the basis of increasingly complex principles; the psychomotor requirements of this test are minimal. On all tasks that required the use of a pencil in concert with visual–spatial analysis and synthesis, she performed at impaired levels. Her graphic renderings of simple and complex visual designs were quite poorly executed, and contained much evidence of visual–spatial distortions.

On the Performance section of the WISC-R, Carla obtained a PIQ of 64. Subtest scaled scores on this section of the WISC-R ranged from a low of 3 on the Object Assembly subtest to a high of 6 on the Block Design subtest. It is apparent that she is suffering from serious deficits in those visual–spatial–organizational skills that this section of the WISC-R was designed to measure.

There were no indications of any simple auditory imperception or suppression with either ear. Performance on a Sweep Hearing Test was not suggestive of hearing impairment.

Carla performed just within normal limits on a test for sound blending and at a moderately impaired level on a test involving the auditory analysis of common words. She performed at a markedly impaired level on a task requiring verbatim memory for sentences of gradually increasing length. She could make no significant progress on a phonemically cued test of verbal fluency.

On the PPVT, Carla obtained a Mental Age of 7 years, 1 month, which is equivalent to an IQ of 111.

On the Verbal section of the WISC-R, she obtained a VIQ of 94. Subtest scaled scores on this section of the WISC-R ranged from a low of 1 on the Digit Span subtest to highs of 10 on the Information, Comprehension, and Vocabulary subtests. It is clear that this girl does not have any marked difficulties in dealing with the type of verbal/linguistic demands involved in the subtests of this section of the WISC-R. Her problems on the Digit Span subtest took the form of perseverative responding.

On the Aphasia Screening Test, Carla made no errors of a clearly aphasic nature. She was well able to follow simple verbal commands and to name pictures of common objects. She was able to name almost all of the letters of the alphabet presented to her. However, there was some evidence of right–left confusion and difficulties in elementary arithmetic calculation.

With much assistance, this girl was able to make some progress on a nonverbal problem-solving task (Category Test, involving elementary concept formation, strategy generation, and the capacity to benefit from positive and negative informational feedback). However, she had considerable difficulty with the age-appropriate strategy-generating and information-processing demands of the test.

On the WRAT-R, Carla was not able to copy all of the simple designs on the Spelling subtest. On the Reading subtest, she identified all but one of the letters of the alphabet presented to her, but could not read any simple words. She did not identify single-digit numerals on a consistent basis. There were some indications that she was capable of elementary conservation of quantity skills, but this was quite inconsistent.

On the PIC (completed by the mother), there were abundantly clear indications that Carla is perceived as suffering from a marked degree of socioemotional disturbance. A combination of internalized and externalized forms of psychopathology may be operative. Similarly, there were clear indications on an activity rating scale and on a behavior problem checklist (both completed by the mother) that Carla is perceived as being afflicted with a significant degree of psychosocial dysfunction.

Neuropsychological Disposition and Implications

Although clearly not diagnostic of any neuropathological condition, this particular pattern of neuropsychological test results would tend to raise some question regarding the functional integrity of Carla's brain. Skills and abilities ordinarily thought to be subserved primarily by some subcortical systems of the brain would appear to be particularly impaired. This profile of neuropsychological test results is largely contraindicative of dysfunction at the level of the cerebral cortex. Rather, disturbance of subcortical structures and systems would be consistent with the clinical picture.

Postscript

We recommended that the parents consult their family physician regarding the advisability of a complete neurological examination of this girl.

We emphasized in both written and oral communications regarding Carla that she did not appear to be making age-appropriate gains in many areas of basic adaptive skills and abilities. Of particular concern were her problems in visual–spatial–organizational skills, psychomotor coordination, and general problem-solving and strategy-generating skills. Her difficulties in modulating her level of arousal to meet changing environmental demands were also very evident.

We expressed particular concern about Carla's progress in dealing with novel material and in generating plans and strategies for dealing effectively with new or otherwise complex situations. In addition, we cautioned parents and other caretakers about her limited capacity to engage in coordinated psychomotor activity, especially under speeded or otherwise complex conditions.

Carla exhibits virtually all of the symptoms and patterns of performance that are associated with the syndrome of NLD. The therapeutic program that we recommend in such cases is presented in Rourke (1989). As has turned out to be the case for Carla, we have found that the institution of this treatment program is particularly effective when begun at relatively early developmental periods. In fact, the earlier the program is begun, the better.

One final note is in order regarding the interaction of neuropsychological assets and deficits on the one hand, and academic and psychosocial functioning on the other. That the program mentioned above can be expected to have a positive impact on both academic and psychosocial functioning is especially comforting to parents and other caretakers. This is the case because these persons are usually of the opinion that academic problems require academic intervention; psychosocial problems, psychosocial intervention; and so on. Demonstrating that these difficulties arise from a common "cause," and that this "cause" can be dealt with therapeutically, is one of the first and most important steps in the exercise of gaining the parents' and other caretakers' cooperation in the implementation of such a program. This is one of the very direct therapeutic benefits that has arisen from the investigation of this particular subtype of LD.

CASE 6: MARY

Relevance

This girl, aged 12 years, 9 months, exhibited a very clear and frequently encountered subtype of LD. Mary had been plagued with failure and frustration within the academic setting since her earliest encounters with it. It was also the case that she did not exhibit any frank psychopathology at the time of her neuropsychological examination. Indeed, except for what appeared to be relatively mild anxiety in some situations, especially surrounding failure at academic tasks and those that she perceived as related to them, she was virtually free of psychosocial disturbance. This case illustrates that a pervasive and rather devastating psycholinguistically based form of LD can be extant over a protracted period of time without any necessary consequences in the form of significant psychosocial disorder.

Our usual quasi-report format is employed to present the results of Mary's neuropsychological examination.

Neuropsychological Assessment Findings

Behavioral Observations during the Examination

Throughout the day-long testing session, Mary was cooperative with the examiner, and rapport was easily obtained and maintained with her. She was attentive to the tasks presented to her. There were no occasions when she exhibited irrelevant motor activity; her general level of psychomotor coordination was average. She exhibited an average amount of verbal interchange with the examiner, and she was socially appropriate. Mary's general demeanor was somewhat reserved, if not taciturn. Her motivation to do well on the tests administered to her was never in any doubt. Although her response speed was, in general, within the average range, there were occasions when she proceeded somewhat quickly on test items.

All things considered, it would appear that a very reliable estimate of Mary's adaptive skills and abilities was obtained in this examination.

Summary of Test Results and Impressions

General Comments. Mary exhibited significant and marked deficits in important aspects of several verbal/linguistic skills within the context of a wide range of other very well-developed adaptive skills and abilities. It is clear that the psycholinguistic deficiencies in evidence would be expected to hamper considerably her attempts at adaptation, including progress within the academic realm. Figure 5.6 presents a summary of Mary's test results.

Test Results and Impressions. There were no indications of any simple tactile imperception or suppression with either hand. Mary experienced no difficulties in identifying symbols written on the fingertips of each hand. There was no clear evidence of finger agnosia or astereognosis for coins with either hand.

On a nonverbal problem-solving task (Tactual Performance Test, involving strategy generation, psychomotor coordination, and the capacity to benefit from tactile input and kinesthetic feedback), her level of performance on a first trial with the right hand was average. Performances on subsequent trials with the left hand and with both hands together were also within normal limits. Mary's incidental memory for the shapes and locations of the blocks used on this task was excellent. It is clear that this type of "hands-on" task constitutes a good learning environment for her; both the input and the output requirements for this task are essentially nonverbal in nature.

Mary would appear to be exclusively right-handed, right-footed, and right-eyed. Strength of grip with the upper extremities and index finger tapping speeds were within normal limits. She experienced much more than ordinary difficulty on a test for foot-tapping speed. There was no clear evidence of any kinetic tremor with the either hand on a test specifically designed for the measurement of this dimension. She performed at a superior level on tests for static steadiness. Speeded eye–hand coordination (Grooved Pegboard Test) was average with the right hand and mildly impaired with the left hand.

There were no clear indications of any simple visual imperception or suppression. Mary performed at an above-average level on a test requiring immediate memory for visual sequences (Target Test).

Mary's graphic renderings of simple visual designs were not marked by significant visual–spatial distortions; however, all yielded some evidence of tremor. Her cursive script was also marked by some tremor. Her drawing of a complex key was quite immature and lacking in visual–spatial detail.

On a task that required the use of a pencil under timed conditions (Underlining Test), Mary experienced some outstanding difficulties. It is notable that she exhibited particular problems on those aspects of this test that involve target and distractor items of a more complex psycholinguistic variety, and on those wherein performance is enhanced through the use of a naming strategy.

Mary obtained a PIQ of 96 on the Performance section of the WISC-R. Subtest scaled scores on this section of the WISC-R ranged from lows of 7 on the Block Design subtest to a high of 12 on the Picture Arrangement subtest. It is clear that she does not exhibit any outstanding deficits in most of the visual–spatial–organizational skills and abilities that these subtests of the WISC-R were designed to measure. The rather minimal verbal requirements of the Block Design subtest may have posed some problems for her.

Mary experienced some difficulty on a task that required her to negotiate a visual–spatial array with a pencil on the basis of the numeric sequence. When this test was rendered somewhat more complex by the addition of the requirement to alternate between the numeric and alphabetic sequences in order to complete the task, her level of performance improved to a normal level. In this and some other instances in this examination, she exhibited a kind of "warm-up" effect: At first she did poorly on the task, but she "recovered" to perform fairly adequately during subsequent phases of it.

FIGURE 5.6. Summary of neuropsychological test results for Case 6 (Mary).

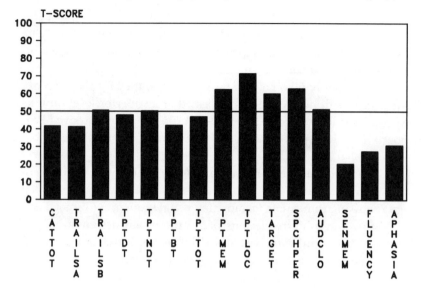

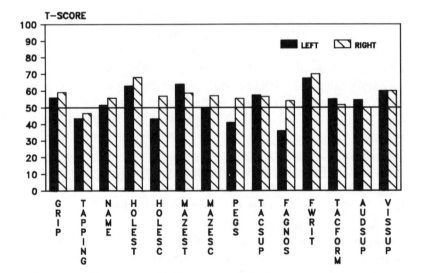

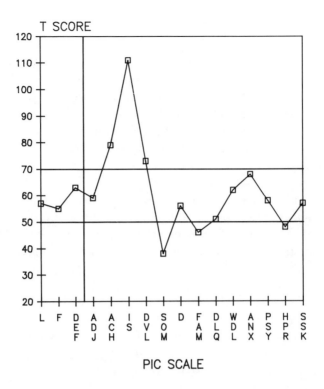

T SCORE

PIC SCALE

Test	Score at 12 yr, 9 mo
WISC-R	
Verbal IQ	73
Information	6
Comprehension	4
Arithmetic	7
Similarities	7
Vocabulary	4
Digit Span	5
Performance IQ	96
Picture Completion	10
Picture Arrangement	12
Block Design	7
Object Assembly	9
Coding	10
Full Scale IQ	83
PPVT IQ	91
WRAT-R	
Reading	75
Spelling	72
Arithmetic	60

There were no indications of any simple auditory imperception or suppression with either ear. Performance on a Sweep Hearing Test was within normal limits. Mary performed very poorly on a task requiring fine auditory discrimination and sustained attentional skills. It is probable that the requirements for both auditory discrimination and sustained attention were problematic for her on this task.

Mary performed at an average level on a test for sound blending. She experienced very marked problems on a test for verbatim memory for sentences and on a phonemically cued test of verbal fluency. Her level of performance was superior on a test that required her to underline the graphic equivalents of novel speech sounds.

On the PPVT, Mary obtained a Mental Age of 11 years, 9 months, which is equivalent to an IQ of 91.

On the Verbal section of the WISC-R, she obtained a VIQ of 73. Subtest scaled scores on this section of the WISC-R ranged from lows of 4 on the Comprehension and Vocabulary subtests to highs of 7 on the Arithmetic and Similarities subtests. These generally depressed scores on this section of the WISC-R reflect her fairly pervasive difficulties in many areas of psycholinguistic development.

On the Aphasia Screening Test, there were no indications of any frank aphasic deficits. However, she experienced considerable difficulty in the enunciation of some complex, multisyllabic words and in simple arithmetic calculation. Problems in the reading and spelling of age-appropriate words were also in evidence.

Performance on a complex nonverbal problem-solving task (Category Test, involving concept formation, strategy generation, and the capacity to benefit from positive and negative informational feedback) was at a borderline level. Mary made some errors on a very elementary subtest of this task that requires reading. Following this very poor level of performance, it is apparent that the provision of immediate feedback regarding the correctness of responses on this test was of considerable assistance to her. However, she still experienced significant difficulties in adapting to this task.

On the WRAT-R, Mary obtained the following approximate grade-equivalent (centile) scores: Reading, 3 (5); Spelling, 3 (3); Arithmetic, 3 (0.8). Many of her misspellings were of the phonetically accurate variety. On the Reading subtest, she attempted to employ a phonetic word attack strategy on some occasions, but her efforts in this respect were largely unsuccessful. Her performance on the Arithmetic subtest suggested that she had not yet mastered many elementary principles relating to basic arithmetic calculation skills. It was also apparent that she misread some arithmetic operation signs and that she could make no progress whatsoever in dealing with common fractions.

On the PIC (completed by her mother), there were no clear indications that Mary was perceived as suffering from any significant degree of socioemotional disturbance. Similarly, there were no clear indications on an activity rating scale and on a behavior problem checklist that she was perceived as exhibiting any significant behavior problems. However, there were some indications on the latter checklist that Mary was perceived as experiencing some anxiety in some isolated situations, primarily of an academic nature.

Neuropsychological Disposition and Implications

Although clearly not diagnostic of any neuropathological condition, this particular pattern of neuropsychological test results would tend to raise some question regarding the functional integrity of Mary's brain. The clinical picture is one that is compatible with long-standing, chronic cerebral dysfunction. Skills and abilities ordinarily thought to be subserved primarily by some systems within the temporal–parietal region of the left cerebral hemisphere would appear to be particularly impaired. It should be emphasized that there is no evidence in this protocol that would be consistent with the presence of any acute neurological disease process.

Mary would be expected to experience considerable difficulty in attempting to learn within a normal or standard academic environment. Those aspects of her psycholinguistic skills that are impaired would appear to pose the principal impediment to progress within such a milieu. The long-term prognosis for habilitation of Mary's deficits would appear to be guarded. With intensive, specialized intervention at this time, there is good reason to believe that some advancement in basic adaptive skills and abilities is indeed probable.

Postscript

At the time of her neuropsychological assessment, Mary did not appear to be afflicted with any type of degree of significant psychopathology. This would appear to reflect the positive aspects of a relatively nurturant and understanding environment at home and at school. However, given the likelihood of continued academic difficulties, we cautioned that this might have some negative implications for her socioemotional well-being.

At the same time, we would emphasize that Mary's virtual freedom from psychosocial dysfunction at the time of the examination demonstrates that severe LD of this nature and psychosocial dysfunction are not inextricably intertwined. Indeed, as was demonstrated in Chapters 2–4 of this volume, it is quite common to find that this is the case.

CASE 7: MICHAEL

Relevance

This 9-year, 1-month-old youngster exhibited a psycholinguistically based variety of LD and no type or degree of psychosocial dysfunction. The case is of particular interest because the language of instruction for Michael (French) was not the same as the language that he used at home and in nonacademic social contexts (English). In such circumstances, we almost always endeavor to introduce the child to a language of instruction that is more in keeping with that employed in the home and social environment. The reason for this is quite simple: Children at this age who have considerable difficulty in dealing with the more basic aspects of language development usually develop academic skills much better in an environment where confusion over words is kept to a minimum. In spite of Michael's marked difficulties with some aspects of linguistic development and an inappropriate educational placement, there was no evidence of psychosocial dysfunction. Indeed, all indications pointed to age-appropriate development within the socioemotional sphere.

Once again, we employ a quasi-report format for the presentation of results. However, in this case, some of the detail evident in previous cases is omitted.

Neuropsychological Assessment Findings

Behavioral Observations during the Examination

Throughout the day-long testing session, Michael was cooperative with the examiner and was reasonably well motivated. He exhibited an average level of general physical activity. He tended to resist guessing at answers about which he was unsure, and there were occasions when he required encouragement to continue with those tasks that he found difficult. There were some indications of impulsivity and distractibility on occasion, but such response styles were not commonplace in his performance repertoire. There were numerous occasions when he seemed at a loss to find words to express himself, and some of his answers to rather simple questions were quite inappropriate with respect to content. There was also some stammering in evidence.

All things considered, it would appear that a fairly reliable estimate of this boy's adaptive skills and abilities was obtained in this examination.

Summary of Test Results and Impressions

General Comments. Michael exhibited a number of deficits in many aspects of psycholinguistic skills. These difficulties and his very apparent problems in maintaining task orientation through verbal means would appear to be at the root of his problems in academic learning. Michael exhibited some very well-developed skills and abilities, mostly of a nonverbal nature. It would appear that he is in need of intensive, specialized assistance if he is to make adequate progress in the academic setting. The following aspects of this report were designed to add some specifications to these generalizations. Figure 5.7 provides a summary of Michael's test results.

FIGURE 5.7. Summary of neuropsychological test results for Case 7 (Michael).

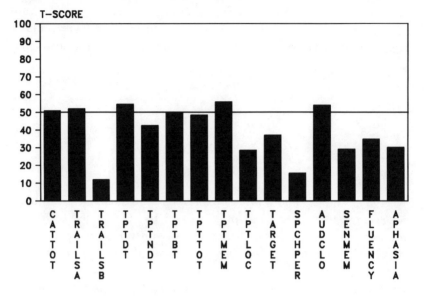

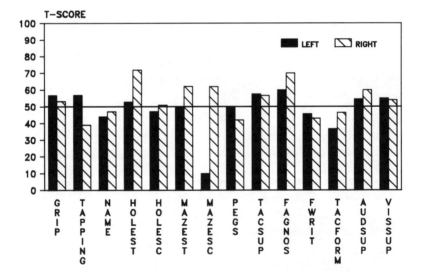

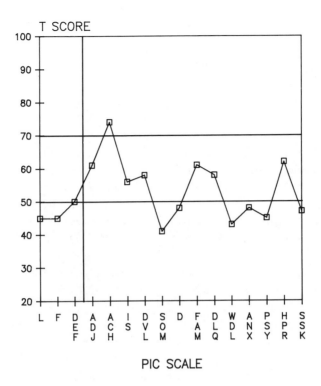

T SCORE

PIC SCALE

Test	Score at 9 yr, 1 mo
WISC-R	
Verbal IQ	91
Information	10
Comprehension	11
Arithmetic	6
Similarities	8
Vocabulary	8
Digit Span	9
Performance IQ	106
Picture Completion	13
Picture Arrangement	13
Block Design	10
Object Assembly	10
Coding	9
Full Scale IQ	98
PPVT IQ	106
WRAT-R	
Reading	55
Spelling	46
Arithmetic	99

Test Results and Impressions. There were no indications of any simple tactile imperception or suppression. A test for finger localization was negative for both hands. Michael experienced some difficulties in identifying coins by touch with each hand; this was more marked with the left hand. He exhibited more than ordinary difficulties in identifying numbers written on the fingertips of the right hand; performance with the left hand was just within normal limits. These tactile–perceptual difficulties may reflect problems in dealing with the symbolic aspects of the material to be identified (coins, numbers), rather than somatosensory deficits per se.

On the Tactual Performance Test, Michael's overall level of performance was quite good. He showed evidence of being able to benefit from the informational feedback provided on this task. However, there were some problems evident in so doing on a second trial with the left hand. His incidental memory for the shapes of the blocks used on this task was average; however, his memory for their proper locations was quite poor. It is probable that the latter problem is reflective of difficulties in the spontaneous verbal coding of information received through the tactile modality.

There were no indications of any simple visual imperception or suppression. He performed at a mildly impaired level on a task designed for the measurement of immediate memory for visual sequences (Target Test). His problems with this test are those usually seen in children of this age who do not spontaneously employ verbal means for the coding of visual information. This can be especially debilitating when the visually presented material to be remembered is presented in a temporal sequence.

On the Performance section of the WISC-R, Michael obtained a PIQ of 106. Subtest scaled scores on the five subtests of this section of the WISC-R ranged from 13 (Picture Completion, Picture Arrangement) to 9 (Coding). It is clear that he is not suffering from any impairment in the visual–spatial–organizational skills and abilities that this section of the WISC-R was designed to measure. However, the symbolic aspects of the Coding subtest may have posed problems for him.

On the Underlining Test (a measure that requires rapid information processing of a variety of verbal and nonverbal target items), Michael's overall level of performance was quite poor. He experienced particular difficulty when he was required to deal with verbal target and distractor items. He missed a very large proportion of the target items on some of the subtests; this is usually seen in youngsters of this age who are having considerable difficulty in maintaining attention and task orientation in situations where verbal direction of behavior is required.

Performance on a task that required him to negotiate a visual–spatial array on the basis of the numeric sequence was within normal limits (Trail Making Test, Part A). However, he exhibited considerable difficulty on another version of this task (Part B) that required him to alternate between the numeric and alphabetic sequences in order to complete the spatial pattern; this is another indication of his difficulty in directing his behavior via verbal means.

Michael would appear to be predominantly right-handed, right-footed, and right-eyed. Strength of grip was average with the right and left hands. Simple motor speed was mildly impaired with the right hand, and average with the left hand. Foot-tapping speeds were impaired, especially with the right foot. There was no evidence of static tremor with either hand. There was no clear evidence of any kinetic tremor with the right hand; however, he did not comply completely with the instructions for this task, thus rendering its interpretation problematic. There was some evidence of tremor with the left hand. Some difficulties in speeded eye–hand coordination were noted with the right hand on a task designed for the measurement of this dimension (Grooved Pegboard Test); left-hand performance on this task was average.

Michael's cursive script was marked by a mild degree of tremor. Tremor was also evident in his graphic reproductions of simple visual designs. There were some very mild visual–spatial distortions evident in his renderings of these designs. He had outstanding difficulties in reproducing the intricate details in a drawing of a key. The latter are often seen in children of this age who experience problems in directing their behavior by verbal means.

There were no indications of any simple auditory imperception or suppression. A Sweep Hearing Test did not reveal any indications of deficiencies in auditory acuity. Michael performed very poorly on a task requiring fine auditory discrimination and sustained attentional capacities (Seashore Rhythm Test). It is notable that the latter task involves attention to nonverbal auditory signals.

On tests designed for the measurement of sound blending and phonemically cued verbal fluency, his levels of performance were average and mildly impaired, respectively. Michael experienced considerable difficulty on a test requiring verbatim memory for sentences of gradually increasing length. It is notable that he was able to grasp the gist of some of the sentences on this task that he could not repeat completely verbatim. His level of performance on a task requiring him to underline the graphic equivalents of novel speech sounds was markedly impaired; his performance was essentially at a chance level on this task.

Michael obtained a VIQ of 91 on the Verbal section of the WISC-R. Subtest scaled scores on this section of the WISC-R ranged from a low of 6 on the Arithmetic subtest to a high of 11 on the Comprehension subtest. This pattern of subtest scaled scores is often seen in children of this age who are experiencing difficulties in psycholinguistic skill development that are hampering their attempts at learning basic academic subjects. Difficulties in maintaining immediate alertness for auditory–verbal messages and in dealing with short bursts of nonredundant verbal information are often characteristic of such youngsters.

On the Aphasia Screening Test, Michael exhibited clear difficulties in the oral and written spelling and reading of age-appropriate words and in the enunciation of complex multisyllabic words. There was one naming error in evidence, and there were several other indications of difficulties in conjuring up words to express himself adequately.

Michael obtained a Mental Age of 10 years, 0 months (equivalent to an IQ of 106) on the PPVT. It is notable that verbal responses are not required on this test.

On the WRAT-R, he obtained the following approximate grade-equivalent (centile) scores: Reading, 1 (0.3); Spelling, <1 (0.03); Arithmetic, 3 (47). Some of Michael's misspellings were of the phonetically accurate variety, but a significant number were not. Most of his reading errors were of the "sight-word/best-guess" variety (e.g., "it" for "eat," "has" for "was," "there" for "then"). It is clear that he experiences considerable difficulty in using a phonetic word attack strategy on a consistent basis for the reading of unfamiliar words. His performance on the Arithmetic subtest was at a roughly age-appropriate level; however, he made a number of errors on relatively simple arithmetic problems. In addition, limitations in memory for arithmetic procedures would appear to have played a role in his difficulties on this subtest.

On a very complex nonverbal problem-solving task (Category Test), his overall level of performance was within normal limits.

His mother's responses on rating scales for hyperactivity and common behavior problems suggested that she did not perceive Michael as susceptible to any significant form or degree of socioemotional disturbance. Furthermore, her responses on the PIC were not suggestive of any type or degree of perceived psychopathology.

Neuropsychological Disposition and Recommendations

Although clearly not diagnostic of any neuropathological disease process, this particular pattern of neuropsychological test results would be compatible with long-term, chronic dysfunction at the level of the cerebral hemispheres. There were no indications in this profile of neuropsychological test results that would be compatible with the presence of any acute neurological disease process. Abilities and skills ordinarily thought to be subserved primarily by the temporal and adjacent frontal and parietal regions of the left cerebral hemisphere would appear to be particularly compromised.

Michael experiences much difficulty in a variety of situations that require him to attend to and assimilate short bursts of nonredundant auditory–verbal information. This sort of demand comes to characterize the academic situation more and more with advancing years. Since he requires much in the way of multimodal, redundant instruction, with an abundance of corrective feedback, in order to make progress in learning, it would appear probable that placement within a "regular" academic milieu would not meet his information-processing needs. Indeed, it would be expected that he would fall further and further behind with respect to academic learning in such a setting. Furthermore, it would appear probable that impulsivity and susceptibility to distraction would be expected to increase therein. Feelings of self-worth and other important socioemotional dimensions of behavior may suffer if his specific information-processing needs are not met in the academic milieu.

It is apparent that Michael has many well-developed skills and abilities, mostly within the nonverbal realm. It is important that the development of these skills and abilities be encouraged and that he come to realize that accomplishments within these areas are valued by those whose opinion he respects. Within the academic milieu, it would seem advisable to encourage such development by accentuating his average to above-average skills and abilities in the projects that are assigned to him.

Michael's problems in directing his behavior by verbal means were especially marked in this examination. This difficulty is not an artifact of the tests being administered in English rather than in French. In view of this significant problem, consideration should be given to placing him in an academic milieu wherein the language of the school would coincide with the one that he speaks with his age-mates and at home. (At the time of testing, this was not the case.)

Postscript

In order to discuss in detail the remedial/treatment ramifications of neuropsychological test results, we routinely meet with parents and those school officials (teachers, principal, educational consultants) who are currently involved with the child. At that time, it is usually possible to formulate a provisional remedial/treatment plan that takes into consideration the facilities and programs that are currently available in the school and the community.

In this instance, we explained in detail the recommendations cited above. Specific issues surrounding graphomotor requirements, preferred learning milieux, and specific remedial programs that might be instituted were discussed. The issue of changing schools so that the language of instruction would match that used in the extra-academic sphere was resolved.

With respect to the issues that constitute the focus of this volume, the principal point to be made in Michael's case is quite simple: Although his psychosocial functioning at the time of this examination was age-appropriate, it could be anticipated that he would continue to fall progressively further behind in his academic work if his specific educational needs were not addressed in an appropriate fashion. Failure to meet these needs would, in the long run, be expected to provoke considerable psychosocial stress and strain for Michael: That is, he could not be expected to be able to maintain psychosocial equilibrium indefinitely in the face of inappropriate attention to his particular educational needs. Once again, we would emphasize that an understanding of the interaction among evolving developmental demands, neuropsychological assets and deficits, and psychosocial functioning is crucial in the clinical management of youngsters with LD.

CASE 8: ROGER

Relevance

The following case illustrates the common, although relatively mild, developmental presentation of the NLD syndrome. The case report is presented in some detail in order to illustrate the dynamics linking this particular subtype of LD to its socioemotional manifestations. The reader may find reference to Case 4 (Jane) instructive with respect to the early manifestations of NLD.

Neuropsychological Assessment Findings

Background

This 47-year-old man was referred for neuropsychological assessment in order to determine the nature and extent of his adaptive skills and abilities. At the time of this assessment, Roger and the referring party were particularly interested in determining which therapeutic/intervention modalities would be beneficial for him.

Behavioral Observations during the Examination

Roger was very cooperative and friendly with the examiner, and rapport was easily obtained and maintained with him. He made eye contact on a consistent basis and engaged in an average amount of verbal interchange with the examiner. He exhibited a somewhat below-average response speed and an average level of general physi-

cal activity. His level of motivation to do well on the tasks administered to him was never in any doubt. There was some evidence of
perseveration of response in problem-solving situations. There were
several occasions when he verbalized aloud his strategies for doing
tests administered to him. All things considered, it would appear
probable that a very reliable estimate of this man's adaptive skills
and abilities was obtained in this examination.

Summary of Test Results and Impressions

General Comments. Roger exhibited a very evident pattern of
relatively impaired visual–spatial–organizational skills, eye–hand
coordination difficulties (more marked on the left side), tactile-
perceptual deficits (more marked on the left side), and higher-level
nonverbal concept formation difficulties; these deficits occurred
within a context of some very well-developed automatic, rote verbal
skills. It should be emphasized that his *levels* of performance in all
but a few isolated (though very important) skill and ability areas
were average to superior. Persons who exhibit this pattern of abilities and deficits are almost always very much at risk for the development of some form of internalized psychopathology—usually
marked by depression, withdrawal, high levels of anxiety, and extreme difficulties in social skills. According to his own and others'
reports, and the examiner's observations of him in the sessions,
Roger would appear to be suffering from these expected effects.

However, it is notable that he appears to be considerably less
anxious than is ordinarily the case with individuals who exhibit
this pattern of adaptive abilities and deficits. Furthermore, his re-
laxed and appropriate interpersonal relations with the examiner are
not typical of such individuals. Such persons usually have much
more difficulty with mechanical arithmetic than with word recognition and spelling; they also have considerable difficulties with concept formation, problem solving, and scientific thinking. All of
these features appear to characterize this man's behavior. The following report was designed to add some specifications to these
generalizations and to offer some suggestions for intervention for
him. Figure 5.8 summarizes Roger's test results.

Test Results and Impressions. There were no indications of any tactile imperception or suppression. There was evidence of finger agnosia with the left hand and borderline indications of finger dysgraphesthesia with the left hand. He exhibited very evident astereognosis for coins with the left hand. Except for borderline finger agnosia, there were no indications of any tactile perceptual difficulties with the right hand.

On the Tactual Performance Test, Roger's overall level of performance was at a borderline level. He did not appear to benefit from continued experience with this task, in that his successive performances on right-, left-, and both-hand trials did not reflect any positive transfer-of-training effect. Performance with the left hand on this test was particularly poor. His incidental memory for the shapes used on this task was at an average level; however, he exhibited much more than expected difficulty in the identification of the proper locations of the blocks on a drawing of the formboard used on this task.

There were no indications of any simple auditory imperception or suppression. Performance on a Sweep Hearing Test suggested that he has a mild to moderate loss in auditory acuity at 8,000 Hz. He performed well within normal limits on a task requiring fine auditory discrimination and sustained attention.

His levels of performance were superior on a test for speech sounds perception. However, performances on tests for sound blending, sentence memory, and phonemically cued verbal fluency were mildly to markedly impaired. His performance on the Sentence Memory Test suggested that he had no difficulties in understanding the gist of sentences that he could not repeat exactly verbatim. It is probable that the deficiencies noted in some of these tasks relate to the fact that English is his second language; it is also possible that his hearing difficulty has a negative impact on the exact hearing of the more difficult sounds of English.

There was no clear evidence of any aphasic deficits on the Aphasia Screening Test.

On the Verbal section of the Wechsler Adult Intelligence Scale (WAIS), Roger obtained a VIQ of 119. Subtest scaled scores on this section of the WAIS ranged from a low of 10 on the Digit Span subtest to a high of 16 on the Arithmetic subtest. It is evident that

FIGURE 5.8. Summary of neuropsychological test results for Case 8 (Roger).

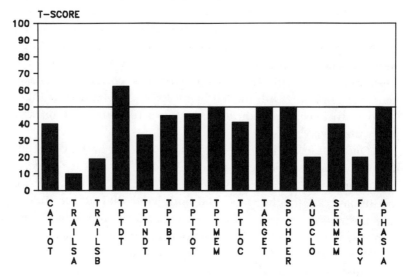

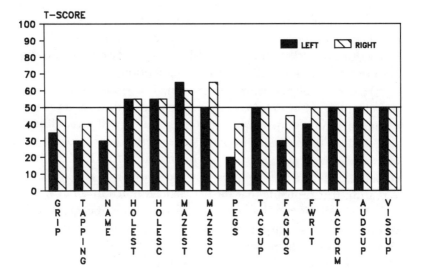

Test	Score at 47 yr, 0 mo
WAIS	
Verbal IQ	119
Information	13
Comprehension	15
Arithmetic	16
Similarities	11
Vocabulary	12
Digit Span	10
Performance IQ	96
Picture Completion	11
Picture Arrangement	7
Block Design	9
Object Assembly	6
Coding	5
Full Scale IQ	109
PPVT IQ	na
WRAT-R	
Reading	105
Spelling	108
Arithmetic	97

the essentially rote verbal requirements of the WAIS Verbal subtests did not pose any problem for him.

There were no indications of any visual imperception or suppression. He performed within normal limits on a task requiring immediate memory for visual sequences (Target Test).

Roger's graphic renderings of simple visual designs were marked by mild visual–spatial distortions and a mild degree of tremor. His graphic rendering of a complex key was somewhat immature and lacking in visual detail. Deficiencies of this sort are often seen in drawings completed by persons who experience considerable difficulty in appreciating and dealing with fine visual detail. His printing was very neat and the letters were very well formed. Cursive script was somewhat less well developed, but certainly quite normal in appearance.

Roger experienced considerable difficulty on a task (Trail Making Test, Part B) that required him to search through a series of numbered and lettered circles, join them together in order, and switch back and forth between the numeric and alphabetic sequence in so doing. This and other observations in the current examination would suggest that he has considerable difficulty in directing his behavior in situations wherein he must deal adaptively with changing task demands. He does much better in situations that require more in the way of straightforward, routinized tasks.

On the Performance section of the WAIS, he obtained a PIQ of 96. Subtest scaled scores on this section of the WAIS ranged from a low of 5 on the Digit Symbol subtest to a high of 11 on the Picture Completion subtest. (It is notable that the Picture Completion subtest is one that is highly correlated with the Verbal subtests of the WAIS.) It is evident that he has difficulties with some aspects of visual–spatial analysis, organization, and synthesis. Ramifications of these difficulties are seen in his problems in generating reasonable inferences regarding cause-and-effect relationships in visual displays of quasi-social relationships; in assembling puzzle parts to form common objects; and in dealing adaptively with a task involving the coordination of symbolic, motor, mnestic, and visual–spatial skills.

Roger would appear to be exclusively right-handed and right-footed, and predominantly right-eyed. Strength of grip was roughly normal with the right hand; that with the left was somewhat impaired. The same situation obtained with respect to finger-tapping speed with each hand. He performed at a superior level on a task specifically designed for the measurement of static steadiness. However, he experienced some mild difficulties on a test for kinetic steadiness. On this task he adopted a slow but accurate strategy, in spite of the instructions to proceed at a much faster pace; this strategy is often employed by persons who are attempting to compensate for some degree of kinetic tremor. His level of performance with the left hand was moderately impaired on a test requiring fine motor coordination under speeded conditions; performance with the right hand on this test was mildly impaired. It is evident that this man experiences increasing difficulty in the motoric sphere as the requirements for eye–hand coordination increase. This difficulty becomes exacerbated dramatically in situations that require the use of the left hand and the integration of information from more than one sensory modality, and/or under speeded conditions.

On a very complex nonverbal concept formation task (involving hypothesis testing, strategy generation, problem solving, and the capacity to benefit from positive and negative informational feedback), Roger's overall level of performance was mildly impaired. His incidental memory for previously correct solutions on this task was somewhat less than expected. There was rather clear evidence of perseveration of response on this test.

On the WRAT-R, he obtained the following approximate grade-equivalent (centile) scores: Reading (word recognition), >12 (63); Spelling, >12 (70); Arithmetic, 8 (42). On the Spelling subtest, virtually all of his misspellings were of the phonetically accurate variety. He also showed himself well able to utilize a phonetic word attack strategy for the decoding of words with which he seemed to be somewhat unfamiliar. Most of his arithmetic calculations were carried out quite systematically; however, there was some inattention to visual detail in evidence, and he did not appear able to deal consistently well with problems involving common fractions. Division involving decimals also posed problems for him. In general, it appeared that he was able to complete successfully those arithmetic problems that involved the application of well-learned verbal rules. However, he experienced considerable difficulty on those problems that required attention to fine visual detail and mathematical reasoning capabilities.

His performances on tests for various aspects of verbal and figural memory were somewhat variable. A test for serial digit learning was performed at a normal level. He performed rather well on the Wechsler Memory Scale (WMS) Logical Memory subtest (a task designed as a measure of verbal memory for meaningful discourse [stories]). His performance on the WMS Visual Reproduction subtest was somewhat poor.

Neuropsychological Disposition and Recommendations

Although clearly not diagnostic of any neuropathological condition, this particular profile of neuropsychological results is often seen in persons of this age who are suffering from significant impairment in skills and abilities ordinarily thought to be sub-served primarily by systems within the right cerebral hemisphere. In addition, subcortical and diffuse white matter dysfunction is often found to be implicated in such cases. This profile would not be consistent with the presence of an acute neurological disease. Rather, this pattern of skills, abilities, and deficiencies is most often seen in persons suffering from a chronic developmental disability that is referred to as the NLD syndrome.

It should be emphasized that the pattern of the manifestations of the NLD syndrome in this man is quite clear, but that the *level* of the deficiencies in evidence in some areas is very mild. In addition, Roger exhibits quite well-developed skills and abilities in areas that are usually quite deficient in individuals who present with this pattern of neuropsychological abilities and deficits.

The treatment program that we have found to be helpful for children and adolescents who present with this neuropsychological profile is outlined in Rourke (1989). Some obvious alterations are necessary in this program in order to adapt it to a man of this age and particular situation.

The ramifications of this particular pattern of abilities and deficits are far-reaching, usually affecting every aspect of voca-tional and social life. Hence, the therapeutic programs necessary to handle these difficulties are always complex and need to be quite comprehensive and integrated. In this connection, it should be pointed out that Roger's own reports of his previous and current socioemotional difficulties are entirely consistent with the mani-festations of internalized psychopathology typical of adults who exhibit the NLD syndrome. However, these are relatively mild in nature, and would suggest that he has had the benefit of very understanding and supporting family, community, and/or special-ized caregivers.

Postscript

One general scenario that often faces persons afflicted with the quality and degree of this man's difficulties is as follows. These remarks are phrased in a general way, and fashioned so as to relate to the expected prognosis in the area of psychosocial functioning for individuals who exhibit the NLD syndrome.

The socioemotional difficulties of persons with NLD appear to result from interactions among and between their neuropsychological assets and deficits. The following are some examples of such interactions:

1. The NLD person's deficits in social judgment would appear to result from more basic problems in reasoning, concept formation, and the like; such problems also lie at the root of their difficulties in mechanical arithmetic and scientific reasoning.

2. Difficulties in visual–spatial–organizational skills are reflected in their problems in identifying and recognizing faces, expressions of emotion, and other subtle nonverbal identifiers of important dimensions of human communication.

3. Lack of prosody, in conjunction with a high volume of verbal output, tends to encourage negative feedback from those who find themselves forced to listen to the seemingly endless recitation of dull, drab, colorless statements that the person with NLD seems impelled to deliver. In a word, the types of speech and language characteristics exhibited by such persons tend to alienate them from others, thus increasing the probability that they will experience socioemotional/adaptational difficulties.

4. Deficits in the tactile–perceptual and psychomotor prowess required for smooth affectional encounters, in conjunction with the NLD person's typically inappropriate judgments regarding nonverbal cues, render intimate encounters all but impossible.

5. Adaptability to novel interpersonal situations is the hallmark of socially appropriate individuals. A combination of aversion for novelty, failure sometimes even to appreciate that an event is in fact novel, and poor problem-solving and hypothesis-testing skills—all of these conspire to render spontaneous, smooth adaptation to the constantly changing milieux of social groups and the interactions inherent therein all but impossible for the NLD individual.

6. Included among the difficulties that arise from limitations in the capacities of the person with NLD for intermodal integration are the following: problems in the assessment of another's emotional state through the integration of information gleaned from

his/her facial expressions, tone of voice, posture, psychomotor patterns, and so on; limitations in the assessment of social cause-and-effect relationships because of a failure to integrate data from a number of sources, such as is often necessary in order to generate reasonable hypotheses regarding the chain of events in social intercourse; failure to appreciate humor because of the complex intermodal judgments required for assessing the juxtaposition of the incongruous; imputing of unreasonable, trite, and/or oversimplified causes for the behavior of others; and imparting such imputations in situations that would lead to embarrassment for the persons so described. These are but a few of the consequences that accrue for the person with NLD because of the difficulties that he/she experiences in integrating information from a variety of sources. Such unfortunate outcomes, of course, are much worse when he/she is anxious and confused (as becomes increasingly common) in novel or otherwise complex situations. It should be clear that such experiences, common as they are for the person with NLD, encourage withdrawal and eventual isolation from social intercourse—with consequences (e.g., depression) that are identical to those proposed above. It should also be clear that this state of affairs increases greatly the probability that individuals so afflicted will feel that others do not wish to be with them; that their behavioral expressions are seen as silly and ridiculous; and that they are powerless in the face of what are for them challenging circumstances (but with which others seemingly deal without difficulty). Thus, it should come as no surprise that depression and suicide attempts occur more frequently than average in individuals who exhibit this syndrome.

It should be emphasized that points 1 through 6 involve interactions between neuropsychological assets and deficits on the one hand and psychosocial difficulties on the other. In Roger's case, as is usual for persons afflicted with NLD, the increasing complexities of developmental demands serve only to worsen their manifestations of socioemotional disturbance. Roger is quite fortunate in that he has at his avail a very solid community support system, which has afforded him many socializing experiences not usually available to most such persons in the North American milieu. Furthermore, he has been assisted considerably by a sensitive psychotherapist who is conversant with the interactions that often transpire in this syndrome.

CASE 9: WILLIAM

Relevance

This case is another illustration of what we refer to as a basic phonological processing disorder (see Rourke, 1989, Ch. 8). The reader should compare this presentation with Case 3 (Chris). In order to illustrate the persistence of this subtype of LD, we present William's test results, which provide longitudinal tracking over almost two decades.

William was first evaluated in middle childhood (9 years, 3 months), was subsequently re-examined 18 months later (10 years, 9 months), and was finally assessed as a young adult (23 years, 11 months). This case is particularly instructive because it demonstrates the relative stability of neuropsychological assets and deficits over the course of development. Moreover, it illustrates the debilitating effects on the acquisition of reading and spelling skills of a rather subtle impairment in the processing of linguistic information. It also serves to demonstrate how a remediational plan that takes into account the individual's adaptive assets and deficits can serve to ameliorate the effects of this particularly intractable type of LD on academic performance.

A Note on Developmental Dynamics

We view the patterns of academic learning experienced by individuals who exhibit this subtype of LD as the direct result of the interaction of specific primary, secondary, tertiary, and linguistic neuropsychological assets and deficits. For example, we would view the primary neuropsychological deficit experienced by this subtype of learning-disabled individuals as having to do with some aspects of auditory perception (principally, exact phonemic hearing). Such a deficit would be expected to eventuate in disordered auditory-verbal attention (secondary deficit); in turn, problems in auditory-verbal memory would be expected to ensue (tertiary deficit). This set of deficits would be expected to eventuate in linguistic deficiencies in areas such as phonological perception, verbal repetition, and so on. The problems in word decoding, verbatim memory for material presented in the classroom situation, and the other deficiencies listed are the expected results of these neuropsychological deficits. We would not anticipate that this set of neuropsychological deficiencies would lead, *in any necessary way,* to problems in socioemotional/adaptive behavior either within or without the academic situation (Rourke, 1988a, 1989).

Summary of Neuropsychological Findings and Implications

Background

William was initially referred for evaluation because of his marked difficulties in the acquisition of basic reading and spelling, despite considerable efforts on the part of both school personnel and parents to assist him. We learned from his grandfather, a pediatrician who was familiar with William's academic problems, that both he (the grandfather) and the boy's father had experienced reading problems in elementary school that persisted until late adolescence. Although it is not always the case, the clinical histories of such individuals often reveal that someone in the immediate family was similarly afflicted.

Test Results, Impressions, Observations

Examination of Figure 5.9 reveals that William's level of psychometric intelligence as measured by the WISC and WAIS was within the normal range over the three assessments. Although it was not evident at the first testing, subsequent evaluations revealed a fairly marked discrepancy between VIQ and PIQ, in favor of the latter. Although it should not be considered a pathognomonic sign, a VIQ–PIQ discrepancy of this magnitude and direction is commonly seen in persons with this subtype of LD.

It is particularly interesting to note that William obtained consistently low scores on the Arithmetic, Digit Span, and Coding (Digit Symbol) subtests, in the context of adequate performances on other measures of verbal and visual–constructional reasoning abilities. We would maintain that these poor subtest performances reflect a relative weakness in the ability to manipulate and deal efficiently with symbolic information. This inference is supported by his relatively deficient performances on the Trail Making Test (Parts A and B), a measure that also appears to require the mental manipulation of symbolic stimuli.

His performance on the Speech-Sounds Perception Test (which requires the identification, in a multiple-choice format, of the graphic counterparts of complex speech sounds) is also instructive. His performances in the first two assessments were particularly poor; by the third evaluation, he performed in an average fashion, relative to normative age cohorts. This latter result was probably a consequence of intensive drill over the years in sound–symbol matching activities. These sorts of "remediational effects" are not unusual in older children and adolescents. It is probably the case that, while such individuals have developed some understanding of simple consonant sound–symbol matching, this skill is not sufficient to produce increased efficiency in the much more complex task of reading (i.e., decoding words). Comparison of the second and third assessments also reveals that William failed to perform effectively on measures involving the blending of speech sounds to form words (Auditory Closure Test) and the generating of words on the basis of phonemic cues (Verbal Fluency Test).

It is evident from inspection of his WRAT scores that William had made very little progress with respect to reading, spelling, and arithmetic over the years. Indeed, even at almost 24 years of age, he had not yet achieved a functional reading level. Not surprisingly, he showed little interest in reading for pleasure; was barely able to read the newspaper; and, in fact, rarely attempted to read unless it was absolutely necessary to do so. William displayed a limited capacity to utilize phonetic encoding and decoding strategies for the purposes of reading and spelling. For example, his misspellings were typically characterized by phonemic omissions and intrusions (e.g., he spelled "educate" as "aucat," "suggestion" as "sudjin," "equipment" as "ecoumant"). This type of qualitative evaluation of spelling errors is often a useful exercise with respect to determining the severity of the person's psycholinguistically based LD (Russell & Rourke, 1991; Sweeney & Rourke, 1978, 1985).

On the positive side, William displayed particular strengths in

FIGURE 5.9. Summary of neuropsychological test results for Case 9 (William).

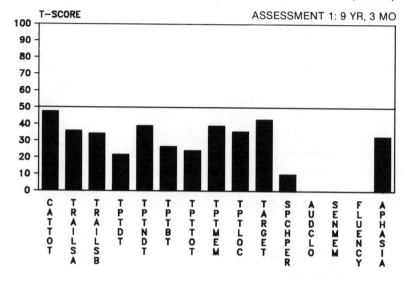

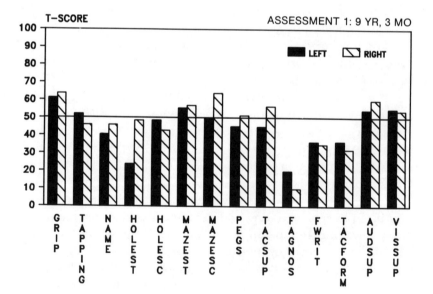

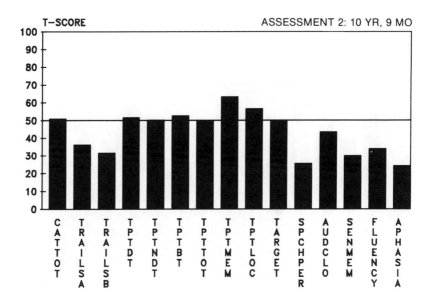

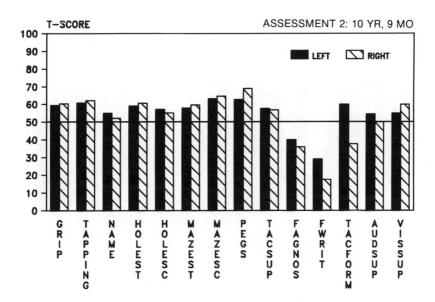

(continued)

FIGURE 5.9. (continued)

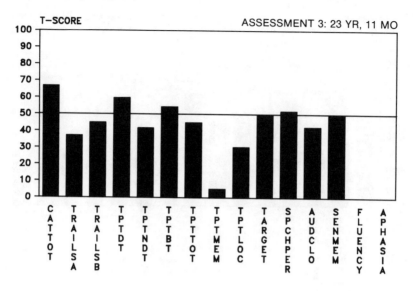

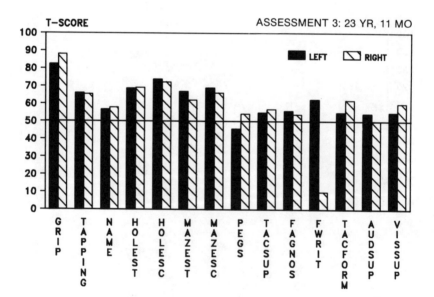

Test	Score at:		
	9 yr, 3 mo	10 yr, 9 mo	23 yr, 11 mo
WISC/WAIS			
Verbal IQ	97	96	97
Information	10	11	9
Comprehension	10	11	12
Arithmetic	7	7	6
Similarities	13	13	13
Vocabulary	12	8	10
Digit Span	5	6	6
Performance IQ	101	121	114
Picture Completion	13	15	11
Picture Arrangement	11	13	12
Block Design	11	14	17
Object Assembly	8	16	13
Coding/Digit Symbol	8	7	8
Full Scale IQ	99	109	104
PPVT IQ	106	107	na
WRAT			
Reading	81	73	66
Spelling	83	73	67
Arithmetic	90	74	77

the visual–motor–organizational skill areas. Indeed, as an adult, he displayed very well-developed simple motor and psychomotor skills, the only exception being low-average performance on the Grooved Pegboard Test with his left hand. His excellent performances on the Category Test in all three evaluations attested to his well-developed nonverbal concept formation and problem-solving skills. Although he experienced some difficulty on the Tactual Performance Test (another measure that involves nonverbal problem solving) in the first assessment, his performances on this test in subsequent evaluations were within normal limits.

Postscript

At the time of the third assessment, William was gainfully employed as a truck driver. He had enroled in a community college upgrading program, and, as subsequent events proved, he was highly motivated to develop his academic skills in order to improve his vocational status. It was also clear from our contacts with him that his family was very supportive. His parents were very sensitive to his limitations in reading, and consequently had not placed unrealistic demands upon him in the academic situation. In view of his emotional stability and obvious motivation to learn, we felt it worthwhile to develop an academic upgrading program utilizing teaching techniques that were based on his neuropsychological strengths and weaknesses.

In order to deliver a remedial educational program for him, we arranged for him to obtain the services of a special education tutor. This particular individual had extensive experience in teaching learning-disabled children and had served as an educational liaison between our clinic and various school boards in the district. Thus, she was familiar with the notion of designing remediational recommendations based on the results of neuropsychological evaluations. We stressed the need for taking advantage of William's visual-motor–constructional and nonverbal problem-solving skills in developing a reading program. Programs were selected that emphasized "word-chunking" techniques, by which William was systematically instructed in identifying morphographs or commonly encountered word chunks (e.g., "ment," "ing"). Although it was often necessary to identify and expand some of the remediational tasks, the emphasis was to name word parts rather than to utilize a phonetic decoding strategy. These procedures were supplemented with sessions in which the tutor would read a passage along with him, followed by gradual fading of the tutor involvement as William was able to read the passage on his own.

The special tutoring program was continued for 2 years, in conjunction with the academic upgrading program at a local community college. At the end of the 2 years, William earned a grade 12 (secondary school) equivalency diploma. His grades in English-language courses were marginal (low C's), but he excelled in mathematics, obtaining grades in the A's in algebra and calculus and grades in the B range in sciences and computer literacy. At the completion of his academic upgrading program, his word recognition skills were estimated to be at roughly a grade 6 level, with reading comprehension in some areas closer to a grade 9 or 10 level. Nevertheless, he felt sufficiently confident to enroll in a preliminary-year university program.

At our most recent contact with William, he was progressing reasonably well in most areas of mathematics. His reading skills are barely sufficient to enable him to keep up with courses that demand more reading than do mathematics courses. He remains eager to learn and is preparing himself for a career in the computer field.

Summary

This case illustrates a number of important characteristics of individuals who suffer from an auditory–verbal type of LD. First, such individuals often display what is best described as a "symbolic" handicap. Their ability to understand spoken language and to express themselves verbally may be quite well developed. However, any task that requires a fine-grained analysis of the phonological structure of words, or places a demand upon the ability to process and manipulate language symbols, is typically quite difficult for them. Furthermore, such persons often display excellent visual and tactile processing capacities within a context of relatively well-developed concept formation abilities and "executive" functioning.

It should be emphasized that the set of neuropsychological assets and deficits described in the previous paragraph would not be expected to hamper William's psychosocial development. In point of fact, this turned out to be the case. Indeed, apart from the vocational limitations imposed by his academic deficiencies, he was performing quite adaptively when we saw him for assessment at the age of almost 24 years.

More generally, serial testing of William over a 14-year span revealed a remarkable stability in his level and configuration of test results, indicating that the underlying neuropsychological assets and deficits of this young man were essentially unchanged. This observation poses a serious challenge to those who would argue that such individuals are merely suffering from a "developmental lag" and that they will eventually "catch up" via maturation and appropriate instruction and remediation. Indeed, our experiences suggest that such individuals suffer from a set of neuropsychological deficits that is typically resistant to remedial strategies designed to attack these weaknesses in a direct fashion.

In formulating a remediational program for William, a number of important factors were taken into account. First of all, William was extremely well motivated and demonstrated a willingness to make exceptional sacrifices in order to improve his academic skills. Second, we were able to formulate a specific teaching method designed to take advantage to his well-developed visual–spatial and nonverbal problem-solving skills. Next, we enlisted the aid of a tutor who was also well motivated and who had considerable experience utilizing neuropsychological test findings in the development of prescriptive programs. Finally, in all of this, William's parents were extremely supportive and, to the best of our knowledge, had never created unrealistic demands for him to achieve in the academic setting. Although obviously the prognosis for continued academic gain must remain guarded, this was in many respects an ideal therapeutic situation. Thus far, rather positive results have been evident for this patient. This is, unfortunately, an outcome that is all too seldom observed in clinical practice, because one or more of the aforementioned elements of this remediational "mix" are frequently absent.

6

Where We've Been and
Where We're Going

A POINT OF VIEW

In this book we have attempted to present a systematic analysis of the relationships that we have found to obtain between psychosocial functioning and learning disabilities (LD). The point of view that emerges from this investigation may be stated as follows:

> Subtypes of LD are manifestations of different patterns of basic neuropsychological assets and deficits. The specific pattern of assets and deficits of any particular subtype of LD may be more or less likely to lead to problems in academic functioning and/or psychosocial functioning. The relationship between neuropsychological assets and deficits, subtypes of LD, and academic and social learning assets and deficits can be understood fully only within a neurodevelopmental framework that takes into consideration the changing nature of the academic, psychosocial, and vocational demands with which humans in a particular society are confronted.

We feel that the research evidence adduced to this point fully supports this rather general view. In addition, we feel that this evidence supports the generalizations and conclusions with which we have ended Chapters 1, 2, 3, and 4.

GENERAL CLINICAL IMPLICATIONS

The case histories presented in Chapter 5 are felt to reflect some of the diversity that is evident among various subtypes of persons with LD. We have also noted the obvious: that the nine cases presented do not exhaust the possibilities that one sees in clinical practice. At the same time, we feel that it is important not to let the idiosyncrasies of this case material blind us to the important dimensions of commonality that obtain within particular subtypes and the very clear differences that obtain between different subtypes. Every clinician aims to treat patients on an individualized basis. However, there is something to be gained from taking into consideration the notion of subtypes, both with respect to LD per se and with respect to the psychosocial problems and difficulties that may accompany them—whether caused by them, or arising from a similar or the same source as the LD themselves. Of the several dimensions of the subtype issue that should be mentioned within this context, many have been addressed in the closing section of Chapter 4 ("Clinical Conclusions").

FUTURE DIRECTIONS

As a result of this review, we see no reason to change our research and model-building program in any significant fashion. However, we do see some important dimensions of the complex interactions with which we have been dealing that require much more investigative effort and much more in the way of expansion and refinement of the conclusions referred to above. These efforts should (and, in our case, will) be directed to the following:

1. The continued specification of the reliability and validity of subtypes of LD and subtypes of psychosocial functioning within the population of children with LD.

2. The continued specification of the relationship between neuropsychological assets and deficits, as manifested in various subtypes of LD in children, and the interaction between these and patterns of normal and abnormal psychosocial functioning.

3. The continued investigation of the developmental dimensions of the interactions mentioned above.

4. Attempts to frame these complex interrelationships within theoretical frameworks that are capable of encompassing their complexity. We feel that a good start has been made with the models presented herein, but that there is much left to do with respect to creative theory and model development in this area.

References

Abelson, A. G., & Mutsch, M. A. (1985). A measure of adaptive behavior of learning disabled students. *Perceptual and Motor Skills, 61,* 862.

Abott, R. C., & Frank, B. E. (1975). A follow-up of LD children in a private special school. *Academic Therapy, 10,* 291–298.

Achenbach, T. M. (1978). The Child Behavior Profile: I. Boys aged 6–11. *Journal of Consulting and Clinical Psychology, 46,* 478–488.

Achenbach, T. M., Conners, C. K., Quay, H. C., Verhulst, F. C., & Howell, C. T. (1989). Replication of empirically derived syndromes as a basis for taxonomy of child/adolescent psychopathology. *Journal of Abnormal Child Psychology, 17,* 299–323.

Achenbach, T. M., & Edelbrock, C. S. (1979). The Child Behavior Profile: II. Boys aged 12–16 and girls aged 6–11 and 12–16. *Journal of Consulting and Clinical Psychology, 47,* 223–233.

Achenbach, T. M., & Edelbrock, C. S. (1981). Behavioral problems and competencies reported by parents of normal and disturbed children aged four to sixteen. *Monographs of the Society for Research in Child Development, 46*(1, Serial No. 188).

Achenbach, T. M., & Edelbrock, C. S. (1983). *Manual for the Child Behavior Checklist and Revised Child Behavior Profile.* Burlington: Department of Psychiatry, University of Vermont.

Ackerman, D., & Howes, C. (1986). Sociometric status and after-school activity of children with learning disabilities. *Journal of Learning Disabilities, 19,* 416–419.

Anderson, S., & Messick, S. (1974). Social competency in young children. *Developmental Psychology, 10,* 282–293.

Applebee, A. N. (1971). Research in reading retardation: Two critical problems. *Journal of Child Psychology and Psychiatry, 12,* 91–113.

Asher, S. R. (1983). Social competence and peer status: Recent advances and future directions. *Child Development, 54,* 1427–1434.

Axelrod, L. (1982). Social perception in learning disabled adolescents. *Journal of Learning Disabilities, 15,* 610–613.

Bachara, G. (1976). Empathy in learning-disabled children. *Perceptual and Motor Skills, 43*, 541–542.

Barkley, R. A. (1981). *Hyperactive children: A handbook for diagnosis and treatment.* New York: Guilford Press.

Barkley, R. A. (1988). Child behavior rating scales and checklists. In M. Rutter, A. H. Tuma, & I. S. Lann (Eds.), *Assessment and diagnosis in child psychopathology* (pp. 113–155). New York: Guilford Press.

Bender, W. N. (1987). Correlates of classroom behavior problems among learning-disabled and nondisabled children in mainstream classes. *Learning Disabilities Quarterly, 10*, 317–324.

Benton, A. L. (1975). Developmental dyslexia: Neurological aspects. In W. J. Friedlander (Ed.), *Advances in neurology* (Vol. 7, pp. 1–41). New York: Raven Press.

Black, F. W. (1974). Self-concept as related to achievement and age in learning-disabled children. *Child Development, 45*, 1137–1140.

Breen, M. J., & Barkley, R. A. (1983). The Personality Inventory for Children (PIC): Its clinical utility with hyperactive children. *Journal of Pediatric Psychology, 8*, 359–386.

Bruck, M. (1987). Social and emotional adjustments of learning-disabled children: A review of the issues. In S. J. Ceci (Ed.), *Handbook of cognitive, social, and neuropsychological aspects of learning disabilities* (Vol. 1, pp. 361–380). Hillsdale, NJ: Erlbaum.

Bruck, M., & Hebert, M. (1982). Correlates of learning-disabled students' peer-interaction patterns. *Learning Disabilities Quarterly, 5*, 353–362.

Bruininks, V. L. (1978a). Actual and perceived peer status of learning disabled students in mainstream programs. *Journal of Special Education, 12*, 51–58.

Bruininks, V. L. (1978b). Peer status and personality characteristics of learning disabled and nondisabled students. *Journal of Learning Disabilities, 11*, 29–34.

Brumback, R. A., & Staton, R. D. (1983). Learning disabilities and childhood depression. *American Journal of Orthopsychiatry, 53*, 269–281.

Bryan, T. (1974a). An observational analysis of classroom behaviors of children with learning disabilities. *Journal of Learning Disabilities, 7*, 26–34.

Bryan, T. (1974b). Peer popularity of learning-disabled children. *Journal of Learning Disabilities, 7*, 621–625.

Bryan, T. (1976). Peer popularity of learning-disabled children: A replication. *Journal of Learning Disabilities, 9*, 307–311.

Bryan, T. (1977). Learning-disabled children's comprehension of nonverbal communication. *Journal of Learning Disabilities, 10*, 501–506.

Bryan, T. (1982). Social skills of learning disabled children and youth: An overview. *Learning Disabilities Quarterly, 5*, 332–333.

Bryan, T., & Bryan, J. H. (1978). *Understanding learning disabilities.* Sherman Oaks, CA: Alfred.

Bryan, T., Donohue, M., & Pearl, R. (1981). Learning-disabled children's communicative competence on referential communication tasks. *Journal of Pediatric Psychology, 6,* 383-393.

Bryan, T., & McGrady, H. J. (1972). Use of a teacher rating scale. *Journal of Learning Disabilities, 5,* 199-206.

Bryan, T., Werner, M., & Pearl, R. (1982). Learning-disabled students' conformity responses to prosocial and antisocial situations. *Learning Disabilities Quarterly, 5,* 344-352.

Bryan, T., & Wheeler, R. (1972). Perception of learning-disabled children: The eye of the observer. *Journal of Learning Disabilities, 5,* 484-488.

Bursuck, W. D. (1983). Sociometric status, behavior ratings, and social knowledge of learning-disabled and low-achieving students. *Learning Disabilities Quarterly, 6,* 329-338.

Camp, B. W., & Bash, M. S. (1981). *Think Aloud: Increasing social and cognitive skills.* Champaign, IL: Research Press.

Capute, A. J., & Accardo, P. J. (1980). The minimal cerebral dysfunction-learning disability syndrome complex. In S. Gabel & M. T. Erikson (Eds.), *Child development and developmental disabilities* (pp. 287-301). Boston: Little, Brown.

Carlson, C. I. (1987). Social interaction goals and strategies of children with learning disabilities. *Journal of Learning Disabilities, 20,* 306-311.

Casey, J. E., Rourke, B. R., & Picard, E. (1991). Syndrome of nonverbal learning disabilities: Age differences in neuropsychological, academic, and socioemotional functioning. *Development and Psychopathology.*

Cerny, L. (1976). Experience in the reeducation of children with dyslexia in Czechoslovakia. *International Journal of Mental Health, 4,* 113-122.

Chapman, J. W. (1988). Cognitive-motivational characteristics and academic achievement of learning-disabled children: A longitudinal study. *Journal of Educational Psychology, 80,* 357-365.

Chapman, J. W., & Boersma, F. J. (1980). *Affective correlates of learning disabilities.* Lisse, The Netherlands: Swets & Zeitlinger.

Chovan, W. L., & Morrison, E. R. (1984). Correlates of self-concept among variant children. *Psychological Reports, 54,* 536-538.

Cohen, M., & Hynd, G. M. (1986). The Conners Teacher Rating Scale: A different factor structure with special education children. *Psychology in the Schools, 23,* 13-23.

Colbert, P., Newman, B., Ney, P., & Young, J. (1982). Learning disabilities as a symptom of depression in children. *Journal of Learning Disabilities, 15,* 333-336.

Conners, C. K. (1969). A teacher rating scale for use in drug studies with children. *American Journal of Psychiatry, 126,* 884-888.

Conners, C. K. (1973). Rating scales for use in drug studies with children. *Psychopharmacology Bulletin* [Special Issue], 24-84.

Cook, T. D., & Campbell, D. T. (1979). *Quasi-experimentation: Design and analysis issues for field settings.* Boston: Houghton Mifflin.

Cooley, E. J., & Ayres, R. R. (1988). Self-concept and success–failure attributions of nonhandicapped students and students with learning disabilities. *Journal of Learning Disabilities, 21,* 174–178.

Cowen, E. L., Pederson, A., Babigian, H., Izzo, L. D., & Trost, M. A. (1973). Long-term follow-up of early detected vulnerable children. *Journal of Consulting and Clinical Psychology, 41,* 438–446.

Cullinan, D., Epstein, M. H., & Dembinski, R. J. (1979). Behavior problems of educationally handicapped and normal pupils. *Journal of Abnormal Child Psychology, 7,* 495–502.

Cullinan, D., Epstein, M. H., & Lloyd, J. (1981). School behavior problems of learning-disabled and normal girls and boys. *Learning Disabilities Quarterly, 4,* 163–169.

Cullinan, D., Schultz, R. M., Epstein, M. H., & Luebke, J. F. (1984). Behavior problems of handicapped adolescent female students. *Journal of Youth and Adolescence, 13,* 57–64.

DeFrancesco, J. J., & Taylor, J. (1985). Dimensions of self-concept in primary and middle school learning disabled and nondisabled students. *Child Study Journal, 15,* 99–105.

DeHorn, A. B., Lachar, D., & Gdowski, C. L. (1979). Profile classification strategies for the Personality Inventory for Children. *Journal of Consulting and Clinical Psychology, 47,* 874–881.

Del Dotto, J. E., Rourke, B. P., McFadden, G. T., & Fisk, J. L. (1987). Developmental analysis of arithmetic-disabled children: Impact on personality adjustment and patterns of adaptive functioning. *Journal of Clinical and Experimental Neuropsychology, 9,* 44. (Abstract)

Denckla, M. B. (1983). The neuropsychology of socioemotional learning disabilities. *Archives of Neurology, 40,* 461–462.

Doll, E. A. (1953). *Vineland Social Maturity Scale.* Minneapolis: Educational Test Bureau.

Dorval, B., McKinney, J. D., & Feagans, L. (1982). Teacher interaction with learning-disabled children and average achievers. *Journal of Pediatric Psychology, 7,* 317–330.

Dudley-Marling, C. C., & Edmiaston, R. (1985). Social status of learning-disabled children and adolescents: A review. *Learning Disabilities Quarterly, 8,* 189–204.

Edgington, R. E. (1975). SLD children: A ten-year follow-up. *Academic Therapy, 11,* 53–64.

Ehrlich, M. I. (1983). Psychofamilial correlates of school disorders. *Journal of School Psychology, 21,* 191–199.

Epstein, M. H., Bursuck, W., & Cullinan, D. (1985). Patterns of behavior problems among the learning disabled: Boys aged 12–18, girls aged 6–11, and girls aged 12–18. *Learning Disabilities Quarterly, 8,* 123–129.

Epstein, M. H., & Cullinan, D. (1984). Behavior problems of mildly handicapped and normal adolescents. *Journal of Clinical Child Psychology, 13,* 33–37.

Epstein, M. H., Cullinan, D., & Bursuck, W. D. (1985). Prevalence of behavior problems among learning-disabled and nonhandicapped students. *Mental Retardation and Learning Disability Bulletin, 13,* 30–39.

Epstein, M. H., Cullinan, D., & Rosemier, R. (1983). Behavior problem patterns among the learning disabled: Boys aged 6–11. *Learning Disabilities Quarterly, 6,* 305–311.

Everitt, B. (1980). *Cluster analysis.* New York: Halsted.

Fafard, M. B., & Haubrich, P. A. (1981). Vocational and social adjustment of learning-disabled young adults: A follow-up study. *Learning Disabilities Quarterly, 4,* 122–130.

Feagans, L., & McKinney, J. D. (1981). The pattern of exceptionality across domains in learning disabled children. *Journal of Applied Developmental Psychology, 1,* 313–328.

Feigin, J., & Meisgeier, C. (1987). Learning disabilities and critical social and behavioral issues: A review. *Journal of Reading, Writing, and Learning Disabilities International, 3,* 259–274.

Fletcher, J. M. (1985). External validation of learning disability typologies. In B. P. Rourke (Ed.), *Neuropsychology of learning disabilities: Essentials of subtype analysis* (pp. 187–211). New York: Guilford Press.

Forbes, G. B. (1987). Personality Inventory for Children: Characteristics of learning disabled children with emotional problems and of emotionally disturbed children with learning problems. *Journal of Clinical Child Psychology, 16,* 133–140.

Fuerst, D. R., Fisk, J. L., & Rourke, B. P. (1989). Psychosocial functioning of learning-disabled children: Replicability of statistically derived subtypes. *Journal of Consulting and Clinical Psychology, 57,* 275–280.

Fuerst, D. R., Fisk, J. L., & Rourke, B. P. (1990). Psychosocial functioning of learning-disabled children: Relations between WISC Verbal IQ–Performance IQ discrepancies and personality subtypes. *Journal of Consulting and Clinical Psychology, 58,* 657–660.

Fuerst, D. R., & Rourke, B. P. (1991a). *Psychosocial functioning of learning-disabled children: Relationships between personality subtypes and achievement test scores.* Manuscript submitted for publication.

Fuerst, D. R., & Rourke, B. P. (1991b). *Patterns of psychosocial functioning of children with LD at three age levels.* Manuscript in preparation.

Gajar, A. H. (1979). Educable mentally retarded, learning disabled, emotionally disturbed: Similarities and differences. *Exceptional Children, 45,* 470–472.

Garrett, M. K., & Crump, W. D. (1980). Peer acceptance, teacher preference, and self-appraisal of social status among learning disabled students. *Learning Disabilities Quarterly, 3,* 42–48.

Gerber, P. J., & Zinkgraf, S. A. (1982). A comparative study of social-perceptual ability in learning-disabled and nonhandicapped students. *Learning Disabilities Quarterly, 5,* 374–378.

Glosser, G., & Koppell, S. (1987). Emotional–behavioral pattern's in children with learning disabilities: Lateralized hemispheric differences. *Journal of Learning Disabilities, 20,* 365–368.

Goh, D. S., Cody, J. J., & Dollinger, S. J. (1984). PIC profiles for learning-disabled and behavior-disordered children. *Journal of Clinical Psychology, 40,* 837–841.

Goldman, R. L., & Hardin, V. B. (1982). The social perception of learning-disabled and non-learning-disabled children. *Exceptional Child, 29,* 57–63.

Green, K. D., Forehand, R., Beck, S. J., & Vosk, B. (1980). An assessment of the relationship among measures of children's social competence, and children's academic achievement. *Child Development, 51,* 1149–1156.

Greenspan, S. (1981). Social competence and handicapped individuals: Practical implications of a proposed model. *Advances in Special Education, 3,* 41–82.

Gresham, F. M., & Elliot, S. N. (1987). Social skill deficits of learning-disabled students: Issues of definition, classification, and assessment. *Journal of Reading, Writing, and Learning Disabilities International, 3,* 131–148.

Hall, C. W., & Richmond, B. O. (1985). Non-verbal communication, self-esteem and interpersonal relations of learning-disabled and non-learning-disabled students. *Exceptional Child, 32,* 87–91.

Hallahan, D. P., Gajar, A. H., Cohen, S. B., & Tarver, S. G. (1978). Selective attention and locus of control in learning-disabled and normal children. *Journal of Learning Disabilities, 11,* 231–236.

Harrington, R. G., & Marks, D. (1985). The Adjustment scale of the PIC as a screening measure for behaviorally disordered children. *Psychological Record, 35,* 465–470.

Harris, J. C., King, S. L., Reifler, J. P., & Rosenberg, L. A. (1984). Emotional and learning disorders in 6–12-year-old boys attending special schools. *Journal of the American Academy of Child Psychiatry, 23,* 431–437.

Healey, K. N. (1987). The price of social ineptitude in learning-disabled children: The challenge ahead. *Journal of Reading, Writing, and Learning Disabilities International, 3,* 149–160.

Hiebert, B., Wong, B., & Hunter, M. (1982). Affective influences on learning-disabled adolescents. *Learning Disabilities Quarterly, 5,* 334–343.

Hisama, T. (1976). Achievement motivation and the locus of control of children with learning disabilities and behavior disorders. *Journal of Learning Disabilities, 9,* 387–392.

Hoge, R. D., & Luce, S. (1979). Predicting academic achievement from classroom behavior. *Review of Educational Research, 49,* 479–496.

Holland, C. J. (1983). *Directive Parental Counseling: The counselor's guide.* Bloomfield Hills, MI: Midwest Professional Publishing.

Horn, W. F., O'Donnell, J. P., & Vitulano, L. A. (1983). Long-term follow-up studies of learning-disabled persons. *Journal of Learning Disabilities, 16,* 542–555.

Hoyle, S. G., & Serafica, F. C. (1988). Peer status of children with and without learning disabilities: A multimethod study. *Learning Disabilities Quarterly, 11,* 322–332.

Jackson, M. A. (1987). The learning-disabled adolescent at risk: Developmental tasks, social competence, and communication effectiveness. *Journal of Reading, Writing, and Learning Disabilities International, 3,* 241–257.

Jacobsen, B., Lowery, B., & DuCette, J. (1986). Attributions of learning-disabled children. *Journal of Educational Psychology, 78,* 59–65.

Jastak, J. F., & Jastak, S. R. (1965). *The Wide Range Achievement Test.* Wilmington, DE: Guidance Associates.

Johnson, D. J., & Blalock, J. W. (Eds.). (1987). *Adults with learning disabilities: Clinical studies.* Orlando FL: Grune & Stratton.

Jorm, A. F., Share, D. L., Matthews, R., & Maclean, R. (1986). Behavior problems in specific reading retarded and general reading backward children: A longitudinal study. *Journal of Child Psychology and Psychiatry, 27,* 33–43.

Keogh, B. K., Tchir, C., & Windeguth-Behn, A. (1974). Teachers' perceptions of educationally high-risk children. *Journal of Learning Disabilities, 7,* 43–50.

Kohn, M., & Rosman, B. L. (1974). Social–emotional, cognitive, and demographic determinants of poor school achievement: Implications for a strategy of intervention. *Journal of Educational Psychology, 66,* 267–276.

Kronick, D. (1980). An overview of research relating to the etiology of interactional deficits in the learning disabled. In R. M. Knights & D. J. Bakker (Eds.), *Treatment of hyperactive and learning disordered children* (pp. 395–407). Baltimore: University Park Press.

LaGreca, A. M. (1981). Social behavior and social perception in learning-disabled children: A review with implications for social skills training. *Journal of Pediatric Psychology, 6,* 395–416.

LaGreca, A. M. (1987). Children with learning disabilities: Interpersonal skills and social competence. *Journal of Reading, Writing, and Learning Disabilities International, 3,* 167–185.

Landau, S., Milich, R., & McFarland, M. (1987). Social status differences among subgroups of learning-disabled boys. *Learning Disabilities Quarterly, 10,* 277–282.

Larson, K. A. (1988). A research review and alternative hypothesis explaining the link between learning disability and delinquency. *Journal of Learning Disabilities, 21,* 357–363–369.

Levin, E. K., Zigmond, N., & Birch, J. W. (1985). A follow-up study of 52 learning-disabled adolescents. *Journal of Learning Disabilities, 18,* 2–7.

Lorr, M. (1983). *Cluster analysis for social scientists.* San Francisco: Jossey-Bass.

Loveland, K. A., Fletcher, J. M., & Bailey, V. (1990). Verbal and nonverbal communication of events in learning-disabled subgroups. *Journal of Clinical and Experimental Neuropsychology, 12,* 433–447.

Margalit, M. (1989). Academic competence and social adjustment of boys with learning disabilities and boys with behavior disorders. *Journal of Learning Disabilities, 22,* 41–45.

Margalit, M., & Zak, I. (1984). Anxiety and self-concept of learning disabled children. *Journal of Learning Disabilities, 17,* 537–539.

Martin, J. S. (1985). *Relationship between sociometric status and social perception in learning-disabled children.* Unpublished doctoral dissertation, University of Georgia.

McCarthy, J. M., & Paraskevopoulos, J. (1969). Behavior patterns of learning-disabled, emotionally disturbed, and average children. *Exceptional Children, 36,* 69–74.

McConaughy, S. H., & Ritter, D. R. (1986). Social competence and behavioral problems of learning-disabled boys aged 6–11. *Journal of Learning Disabilities, 19,* 39–45.

McGee, R., Williams, S., Share, D. L., Anderson, J., & Silva, P. A. (1986). The relationship between specific reading retardation, general reading backwardness, and behavioural problems in a large sample of Dunedin boys: A longitudinal study from five to eleven years. *Journal of Child Psychology and Psychiatry, 27,* 597–610.

McKinney, J. D. (1989). Longitudinal research on the behavioral characteristics of children with learning disabilities. *Journal of Learning Disabilities, 22,* 141–150, 165.

McKinney, J. D., Mason, J., Perkerson, K., Clifford, M. (1975). Relationship between classroom behavior and academic achievement. *Journal of Educational Psychology, 67,* 198–203.

McKinney, J. D., Short, E. J., & Feagans, L. (1985). Academic consequences of perceptual–linguistic subtypes of learning-disabled children. *Learning Disabilities Research, 1,* 6–17.

McKinney, J. D., & Speece, D. L. (1983). Classroom behavior and the academic progress of learning-disabled students. *Journal of Applied Developmental Psychology, 4,* 149–161.

McKinney, J. D., & Speece, D. L. (1986). Academic consequences and longitudinal stability of behavioral subtypes of learning-disabled children. *Journal of Educational Psychology, 78,* 365–372.

Morris, R., Blashfield, R., & Satz, P. (1981). Neuropsychology and cluster analysis: Potentials and problems. *Journal of Clinical Neuropsychology, 3,* 79–99.

Morris, R., Blashfield, R., & Satz, P. (1986). Developmental classification of reading-disabled children. *Journal of Clinical and Experimental Neuropsychology, 8,* 371–392.

Nakamura, C. Y., & Finck, D. N. (1980). Relative effectiveness of socially oriented and task-oriented children and predictability of their behaviors. *Monographs of the Society for Research in Child Development, 45*(3–4, Serial No. 185).

Nussbaum, N. L., & Bigler, E. D. (1986). Neuropsychological and behavioral profiles of empirically derived subgroups of learning-disabled children. *International Journal of Clinical Neuropsychology, 8,* 82–89.

Nussbaum, N. L., Bigler, E. D., Koch, W. R., Ingram, W., Rosa, L., & Massman, P. (1988). Personality/behavioral characteristics in children: Differential effects of putative anterior versus posterior cerebral asymmetry. *Archives of Clinical Neuropsychology, 3,* 127–135.

Owen, F. W., Adams, P. A., Forrest, T., Stolz, L. M., & Fisher, S. (1971). Learning disorders in children: Sibling studies. *Monographs of the Society for Research in Child Development, 36*(4, Serial No. 144).

Ozols, E. J., & Rourke, B. P. (1985). Dimensions of social sensitivity in two types of learning-disabled children. In B. P. Rourke (Ed.), *Neuropsychology of learning disabilities: Essentials of subtype analysis* (pp. 281–301). New York: Guilford Press.

Ozols, E. J., & Rourke, B. P. (1988). Characteristics of young learning-disabled children classified according to patterns of academic achievement: Auditory–perceptual and visual–perceptual abilities. *Journal of Clinical Child Psychology, 17,* 44–52.

Pearl, R., & Cosden, M. (1982). Sizing up a situation: Learning-disabled children's understanding of social interactions. *Learning Disabilities Quarterly, 5,* 371–373.

Perlmutter, B. F., Crocker, J., Cordray, D., & Garstecki, D. (1983). Sociometric status and related personality characteristics of mainstreamed learning-disabled adolescents. *Learning Disabilities Quarterly, 5,* 371–373.

Pickar, D. B. (1986). Psychosocial aspects of learning disabilities: A review of research. *Bulletin of the Menninger Clinic, 50,* 22–32.

Pickar, D. B., & Tori, C. D. (1986). The learning-disabled adolescent: Eriksonian psychosocial development, self-concept, and delinquent behavior. *Journal of Youth and Adolescence, 15,* 429–440.

Porter, J., & Rourke, B. P. (1985). Socioemotional functioning of learning-disabled children: A subtypal analysis of personality patterns. In B. P. Rourke (Ed.), *Neuropsychology of learning disabilities: Essentials of subtype analysis* (pp. 257–279). New York: Guilford Press.

Quay, H. C., & Peterson, D. R. (1975). *Manual for the Behavior Problem Checklist.* Unpublished manuscript, University of Miami.

Raskind, M. H., Drew, D. E., & Regan, J. O. (1983). Nonverbal communication signals in behavior-disordered and non-disordered learning-disabled boys and non-learning-disabled boys. *Learning Disabilities Quarterly, 6,* 12–19.

Raven, J. C. (1960). *Guide to the Standard Progressive Matrices.* London: H. K. Lewis.

Richey, D. D., & McKinney, J. D. (1978). Classroom behavioral styles of learning-disabled boys. *Journal of Learning Disabilities, 11,* 297–302.

Richmond, B. O., & Blagg, D. E. (1985). Adaptive behavior, social adjustment, and academic achievement of regular and special education children. *Exceptional Child, 32,* 93–98.

Rothstein, A., Benjamin, L., Crosby, M., & Eisenstadt, K. (1988). *Learning disorders: An integration of neuropsychological and psychoanalytic considerations.* Madison, CT: International Universities Press.

Rourke, B. P. (1975). Brain–behavior relationships in children with learning disabilities. *American Psychologist, 30,* 911–920.

Rourke, B. P. (1976). Reading retardation in children: Developmental lag or deficit? In R. M. Knights & D. J. Bakker (Eds.), *Neuropsychology of learning disorders: Theoretical approaches* (pp. 125–137). Baltimore: University Park Press.

Rourke, B. P. (1978a). Neuropsychological research in reading retardation: A review. In A. L. Benton & D. Pearl (Eds.), *Dyslexia: An appraisal of current knowledge* (pp. 141–171). New York: Oxford University Press.

Rourke, B. P. (1978b). Reading, spelling, arithmetic disabilities: A neuropsychologic perspective. In H. R. Myklebust (Ed.), *Progress in learning disabilities* (Vol. 4, pp. 97–120). New York: Grune & Stratton.

Rourke, B. P. (1982). Central processing deficiencies in children: Toward a developmental neuropsychological model. *Journal of Clinical Neuropsychology, 4,* 1–18.

Rourke, B. P. (1983). Reading and spelling disabilities: A developmental neuropsychological perspective. In U. Kirk (Ed.), *Neuropsychology of language, reading, and spelling* (pp. 209–234). New York: Academic Press.

Rourke, B. P. (Ed.). (1985). *Neuropsychology of learning disabilities: Essentials of subtype analysis.* New York: Guilford Press.

Rourke, B. P. (1987). Syndrome of nonverbal learning disabilities: The final common pathway of white-matter disease/dysfunction? *Clinical Neuropsychologist, 1,* 209–234.

Rourke, B. P. (1988a). Socioemotional disturbances of learning-disabled children. *Journal of Consulting and Clinical Psychology, 56,* 801–810.

Rourke, B. P. (1988b). The syndrome of nonverbal learning disabilities: Developmental manifestations in neurological disease, disorder, and dysfunction. *Clinical Neuropsychologist, 2,* 293–330.

Rourke, B. P. (1989). *Nonverbal learning disabilities: The syndrome and the model.* New York: Guilford Press.

Rourke, B. P. (Ed.). (1991). *Neuropsychological validation of learning disability subtypes.* New York: Guilford Press.

Rourke, B. P., Bakker, D. J., Fisk, J. L., & Strang, J. D. (1983). *Child neuropsychology: An introduction to theory, research, and clinical practice.* New York: Guilford Press.

Rourke, B. P., Del Dotto, J. E., Rourke, S. B., & Casey, J. E. (1990). Nonverbal learning disabilities: The syndrome and a case study. *Journal of School Psychology, 28,* 361–385.

Rourke, B. P., Dietrich, D. M., & Young, G. C. (1973). Significance of WISC Verbal–Performance discrepancies for younger children with learning disabilities. *Perceptual and Motor Skills, 36,* 275–282.

Rourke, B. P., & Finlayson, M. A. J. (1978). Neuropsychological significance of variations in patterns of academic performance: Verbal and visual–spatial abilities. *Journal of Abnormal Child Psychology, 6,* 121–133.

Rourke, B. P., & Fisk, J. L. (1981). Socioemotional disturbances of learning disabled children: The role of central processing deficits. *Bulletin of the Orton Society, 31,* 77–88.

Rourke, B. P., & Fisk, J. L. (1988). Subtypes of learning-disabled children: Implications for a neurodevelopmental model of differential hemispheric processing. In D. L. Molfese & S. J. Segalowitz (Eds.), *Brain lateralization in children: Developmental implications* (pp. 547–565). New York: Guilford Press.

Rourke, B. P., Fisk, J. L., & Strang, J. D. (1986). *Neuropsychological assessment of children: A treatment-oriented approach.* New York: Guilford Press.

Rourke, B. P., & Strang, J. D. (1978). Neuropsychological significance of variations in patterns of academic performance: Motor, psychomotor, and tactile-perceptual abilities. *Journal of Pediatric Psychology, 3,* 62–66.

Rourke, B. P., & Strang, J. D. (1983). Subtypes of reading and arithmetical disabilities: A neuropsychological analysis. In M. Rutter (Ed.), *Developmental neuropsychiatry* (pp. 473–488). New York: Guilford Press.

Rourke, B. P., & Telegdy, G. A. (1971). Lateralizing significance of WISC Verbal–Performance discrepancies for older children with learning disabilities. *Perceptual and Motor Skills, 33,* 875–883.

Rourke, B. P., Young, G. C., & Flewelling, R. W. (1971). The relationships between WISC Verbal–Performance discrepancies and selected verbal, auditory–perceptual, visual–perceptual, and problem-solving abilities in children with learning disabilities. *Journal of Clinical Psychology, 27,* 475–479.

Rourke, B. P., Young, G. C., Strang, J. D., & Russell, D. L. (1986). Adult outcomes of central processing deficiencies in childhood. In I. Grant & K. M. Adams (Eds.), *Neuropsychological assessment in neuropsychiatric disorders: Clinical methods and empirical findings* (pp. 244–267). New York: Oxford University Press.

Russell, D. L., & Rourke, B. P. (1991). Concurrent and predictive validity of phonetic accuracy of misspellings in normal and disabled readers and spellers. In B. P. Rourke (Ed.), *Neuropsychological validation of learning disability subtypes* (pp. 57–71). New York: Guilford Press.

Sabatino, D. A. (1982). Research on achievement motivation with learning-disabled populations. *Advances in Learning and Behavioral Disabilities, 1,* 75–116.

Sabornie, E. J., & Kauffman, J. M. (1986). Social acceptance of learning-disabled adolescents. *Learning Disabilities Quarterly, 9,* 55–60.

Sainato, D. M., Zigmond, N., & Strain, P. S. (1983). Social status and initiations of interaction by learning-disabled students in a regular education setting. *Analysis and Intervention in Developmental Disabilities, 3,* 71–87.

Schaefer, E. S., Edgerton, M., & Aronson, M. (1977). *Classroom Behavior Inventory.* Chapel Hill, NC: Frank Porter Graham Child Development Center.

Schumaker, J. B., & Hazel, J. S. (1984). Social skills assessment and training for the learning disabled: Who's on first and what's on second. *Journal of Learning Disabilities, 17,* 422–431.

Schumaker, J. B., Hazel, J. S., Sherman, J. A., & Sheldon, J. (1982). Social skill performances of learning-disabled, non-learning disabled, and delinquent adolescents. *Learning Disabilities Quarterly, 5,* 388–397.

Scranton, T. R., & Ryckman, D. B. (1979). Sociometric status of learning-disabled children in an integrative program. *Journal of Learning Disabilities, 12,* 402–407.

Shirer, C., Wiener, J., & Harris, P. J. (1988, June). Academic achievement, social behaviour and correlates of peer status in learning disabled children. In J. Wiener (Chair), *Correlates of peer status in learning-disabled children.* Symposium conducted at the annual meeting of the Canadian Psychological Association, Montreal.

Siegel, E. (1974). *The exceptional child grows up.* New York: E. P. Dutton.

Silver, D. S., & Young, R. D. (1985). Interpersonal problem-solving abilities, peer status, and behavioral adjustment in learning-disabled and non-learning-disabled adolescents. *Advances in Learning and Behavioral Disabilities, 4,* 201–223.

Silverman, R., & Zigmond, N. (1983). Self-concept in learning-disabled adolescents. *Journal of Learning Disabilities, 16,* 478–482.

Siperstein, G. N., Bopp, M. J., & Bak, J. J. (1978). Social status of learning-disabled children. *Journal of Learning Disabilities, 11,* 98–102.

Siperstein, G. N., & Goding, M. J. (1983). Social integration of learning-disabled children in regular classrooms. *Advances in Learning and Behavioral Disabilities, 2,* 227–263.

Sobol, M. P., Earn, B. M., Bennett, D., & Humphries, T. (1983). A categorical analysis of the social attributions of learning-disabled children. *Journal of Abnormal Child Psychology, 11,* 217–228.

Sparrow, S. S., Balla, D. A., & Cicchetti, D. V. (1984). *The Vineland Adaptive Behavior Scales: A revision of the Vineland Social Maturity Scale by Edgar A. Doll.* Circle Pines, MN: American Guidance Services.

Speece, D. L., McKinney, J. D., & Appelbaum, M. I. (1985). Classification and validation of behavioral subtypes of learning-disabled children. *Journal of Educational Psychology, 77,* 67–77.

Sprafkin, J., & Gadow, K. D. (1987). An observational study of emotionally disturbed and learning-disabled children in school settings. *Journal of Abnormal Child Psychology, 15,* 393–408.

Spreen, O. (1988). *Learning-disabled children growing up: A follow-up into adulthood.* New York: Oxford University Press.

Spreen, O. (1989). The relationship between learning disabilities, emotional disorders, and neuropsychology: Some results and observations. *Journal of Clinical and Experimental Neuropsychology, 11,* 117–140.

Stellern, J., Marlowe, M., Jacobs, J., & Cossairt, A. (1985). Neuropsychological significance of right hemisphere cognitive mode in behavior disorders. *Behavioral Disorders, 2,* 113–124.

Stephens, V., Wiener, J., & Harris, P. J. (1988, June). The relationship between special education placement and peer status in learning-disabled children. In J. Wiener (Chair), *Correlates of peer status in learning-disabled children.* Symposium conducted at the annual meeting of the Canadian Psychological Association, Montreal.

Stiliadis, K., & Wiener, J. (in press). Relationship between social perception and peer status in children with learning disabilities. *Journal of Learning Disabilities.*

Stone, W. L., & LaGreca, A. N. (1984). Comprehension of nonverbal communication: A reexamination of the social competencies of learning-disabled children. *Journal of Abnormal Child Psychology, 12,* 505–518.

Strang, J. D. (1981). *Personality dimensions of learning-disabled children: Age and subtype differences.* Unpublished doctoral dissertation, University of Windsor.

Strang, J. D., & Rourke, B. P. (1983). Concept-formation/nonverbal reasoning abilities of children who exhibit specific academic problems with arithmetic. *Journal of Clinical Child Psychology, 12,* 33–39.

Strang, J. D., & Rourke, B. P. (1985a). Adaptive behavior of children with specific arithmetic disabilities and associated neuropsychological abilities and deficits. In B. P. Rourke (Ed.), *Neuropsychology of learning disabilities: Essentials of subtype analysis* (pp. 302–328). New York: Guilford Press.

Strang, J. D., & Rourke, B. P. (1985b). Arithmetic disability subtypes: The neuropsychological significance of specific arithmetical impairment in childhood. In B. P. Rourke (Ed.), *Neuropsychology of learning disabilities: Essentials of subtype analysis* (pp. 167–183). New York: Guilford Press.

Sturge, C. (1982). Reading retardation and antisocial behavior. *Journal of Child Psychology and Psychiatry, 23,* 21-31.

Sweeney, J. E., & Rourke, B. P. (1978). Neuropsychological significance of phonetically accurate and phonetically inaccurate spelling errors in younger and older retarded spellers. *Brain and Language, 5,* 212-225.

Sweeney, J. E., & Rourke, B. P. (1985). Spelling disability subtypes. In B. P. Rourke (Ed.), *Neuropsychology of learning disabilities: Essentials of subtype analysis* (pp. 147-166). New York: Guilford Press.

Tarver, S. G., & Hallahan, D. P. (1974). Attention deficits in children with learning disabilities: A review. *Journal of Learning Disabilities, 7,* 560-569.

Thomas, A. (197 9). Learned helplessness and expectancy factors: Implications for research in learning disabilities. *Review of Educational Research, 49,* 208-221.

Tramontana, M. G. (1983). Neuropsychological evaluation of children and adolescents with psychopathological disorders. In C. J. Golden & P. J. Vicente (Eds.), *Foundations of clinical neuropsychology* (pp. 309-340). New York: Plenum.

Tramontana, M. G., Hooper, S. R., & Nardolillo, E. M. (1988). Behavioral manifestations of neuropsychological impairment in children with psychiatric disorders. *Archives of Clinical Neuropsychology, 3,* 369-374.

Tramontana, M. G., & Sherrets, S. D. (1985). Brain impairment in child psychiatric disorders: Correspondencies between neuropsychological and CT scan results. *Journal of the American Academy of Child Psychiatry, 24,* 590-596.

Tramontana, M. G., Sherrets, S. D., & Golden, C. J. (1980). Brain dysfunction in youngsters with psychiatric disorders: Application of Selz-Reitan rules for neuropsychological diagnosis. *Clinical Neuropsychology, 2,* 118-123.

Wallander, J. L., & Hubert, N. C. (1987). Peer social dysfunction in children with developmental disabilities: Empirical basis and a conceptual model. *Clinical Psychology Review, 7,* 205-221.

Wechsler, D. (1949). *Wechsler Intelligence Scale for Children.* New York: Psychological Corporation.

Wechsler, D. (1974). *Wechsler Intelligence Scale for Children—Revised.* New York: Psychological Corporation.

Weintraub, S., & Mesulam, M. M. (1983). Developmental learning disability of the right hemisphere: Emotional, interpersonal, and cognitive components. *Archives of Neurology, 40,* 463-468.

Weiss, E. (1984). Learning-disabled children's understanding of social interactions of peers. *Journal of Learning Disabilities, 17,* 612-615.

Weller, C., & Strawser, S. (1987). Adaptive behavior of subtypes of learning-disabled individuals. *Journal of Special Education, 21,* 101-115.

Weller, C., Strawser, S., & Buchanan, M. (1985). Adaptive behavior: Designator of a continuum of severity of learning-disabled individuals. *Journal of Learning Disabilities, 18,* 200–204.

Werner, E. E., & Smith, R. S. (1979). An epidemiologic perspective on some antecedents and consequences of childhood mental health problems and learning disabilities: A report from the Kauai longitudinal study. *Journal of the American Academy of Child Psychiatry, 18,* 292–306.

Wiener, J. (1980). A theoretical model of the acquisition of peer relationships of learning-disabled children. *Journal of Learning Disabilities, 13,* 42–47.

Weiner, J. (1987). Peer status of learning-disabled children and adolescents: A review of the literature. *Learning Disabilities Research, 2,* 62–79.

Wiig, E. H., & Harris. S. P. (1974). Perception and interpretation of nonverbally expressed emotions by adolescents with learning disabilities. *Perceptual and Motor Skills, 38,* 239–245.

Wilgosh, L., & Paitich, D. (1982). Delinquency and learning disabilities. *Journal of Learning Disabilities, 15,* 278–279.

Winne, P. H., Woodlands, M. J., & Wong, B. Y. L. (1982). Comparability of self-concept among learning-disabled, normal, and gifted students. *Journal of Learning Disabilities, 15,* 470–475.

Wirt, R. D., Lachar, D., Klinedinst, J. K., & Seat, P. D. (1977). *Multidimensional description of child personality: A manual for the Personality Inventory for Children.* Los Angeles: Western Psychological Services.

Wirt, R. D., Lachar, D., Klinedinst, J. K., & Seat, P. D. (1984). *Multidimensional description of child personality: A manual for the Personality Inventory for Children—Revised 1984.* Los Angeles: Western Psychological Services.

Zimmerman, I. L., & Allebrand, G. N. (1965). Personality characteristics and attitudes toward achievement of good and poor readers. *Journal of Educational Research, 57,* 28–30.

Index

Antisocial behavior, 12–14, 19, 20, 40, 86
Anxiety, 6, 11, 12, 29, 30, 40, 49, 52, 65–67, 70, 71, 139, 156
Attention deficit, 8, 18, 40, 51, 100
case study, 101–108
Attributions, 32–37
developmental considerations, 34–36
and learned helplessness, 33, 34, 36, 87
relationship to aberrant behavior, 35, 36
Autistic behavior, 20

B

Basic phonological processing disorder
case studies, 109–117, 165–174
developmental dynamics, 165, 166

C

Checklists
Behavior Problem Checklist, 9–12, 40
Child Behavior Checklist, 13, 71
Cluster analysis, 41, 50–53, 55

Conclusions
clinical, 86, 87
principal, 85
Conduct problems, 8–13, 18, 40, 41, 52, 65, 78
case study, 91–101

D

Delinquent behavior (*see* Antisocial behavior)
Depression, 5, 11, 20, 49, 52, 65, 66, 70, 81, 156, 164
Developmental dynamics, 165, 166

F

Factor analysis
Q-type, 39, 40, 48–51
R-type, 39, 40
Future directions, 176, 177

H

Heterogeneity, 39–41 (*see also* Psychosocial subtypes; Windsor Taxonomic Research)

Heterogeneity (*continued*)
  methodological considerations,
    39, 48
Hyperactivity, 8, 18, 40, 51, 52, 58,
    59, 65, 71
Hypothesis *1*, 4-6
  case study, 101-109
  definition, 4
Hypothesis *2*, 6-47, 67
  definition, 6
Hypothesis *3*, 69-85
  case studies, 117-131, 131-
    139
  definition, 69

I

Inventories (*see also* Personality
    Inventory for Children)
  Classroom Behavior Inventory,
    41
  MMPI, 20

L

Learning disabilities subtypes, 39,
    44-47 (*see also* Basic
    phonological processing
    disorder; Nonverbal
    learning disabilities)
  circumscribed psycholinguistic
    deficits (case studies), 139-
    146, 146-155
  Group A and Group R-S, 44-47,
    72-74, 80, 82
  "output" (case study), 91-101
  and psychosocial functioning,
    73, 74, 80, 82
Locus of control (*see* Attributions)
Longitudinal studies, 16-20, 41

M

Methodological considerations, 37-
    39, 43, 44 (*see also*
    Heterogeneity; Social
    competence)
  definition of learning
    disabilities, 38
  developmental considerations,
    38, 71, 72
  measurement of maladjustment,
    38

N

Nonverbal learning disabilities (*see
    also* Learning disabilities
    subtypes, Group A)
  adult presentation, 80, 81, 155-
    164
  description and model of, 83, 84
  developmental presentation (case
    studies), 117-131, 155-164
  early manifestations (case study),
    131-139
  and psychopathology, 82-84
  and social competence, 162-164

O

Observation
  of classroom behavior, 8, 9
  of teacher interactions, 26, 27

P

Personality Inventory for Children
    (*see also* Psychosocial

subtypes; Windsor Taxonomic Research)
learning-disabled children versus behavior-disordered children, 15, 16
nonverbal learning disabilities profile, 84
use as a screening device, 15
Psychiatric populations
CT abnormalities, 81
methodological problems, 81
patterns of neuropsychological impairment, 81
Psychosocial subtypes, 39–41, 48–68 (*see also* Windsor Taxonomic Research)
Conduct Disorder, 52, 54, 59, 65
Externalized Psychopathology, 49–54, 58, 66
Internalized Psychopathology, 49–54, 58, 66
Mild Anxiety, 52, 54, 58, 59, 65
Mild Hyperactive, 51, 52, 54, 59, 65
Normal, 49–54, 58, 61, 65
relationship with age, 41, 66, 67
relationships with cognitive and academic functioning, 78–80
Somatic Concern, 49, 52, 54, 59, 65

R

Rating scales (*see also* Checklists)
Conners Teacher Rating Scale, 13
Vineland Adaptive Behavior Scales, 129, 130
Vineland Social Maturity Scale, 127
Remediation (*see* Treatment)

S

Self-esteem/self-concept, 28–32, 34–37, 87, 116, 153, 164
and attributions, 34
developmental considerations, 34–36
effect of socioeconomic status, 31
relationship to aberrant behavior, 35, 36
Social competence, 41–47
components of, 42
methodological considerations, 43, 44
and neuropsychological functioning, 44–47, 163, 164
single-deficit hypotheses, 43
Social networks, 25, 26
Social status, 20–28, 87
nomination techniques, 21–23, 25
rating scales, 23–26
self-perception of, 24, 26
with teachers, 26, 27
Suicide, 164

T

Treatment
guidelines, 86–89
examples, 92, 100, 101, 108, 109, 117, 125–129, 132, 138, 139, 153–155, 162, 172–174

V

Verbal IQ–Performance IQ discrepancies, 23, 74–76, 79–81

W

Windsor Taxonomic Research, 48–
68 (*see also* Heterogeneity;
Psychosocial subtypes)
description of the typology, 60–
66

development of the typology,
49–54
internal validity, 54–59
relationship with age, 66–68
relationship with WISC VIQ-
PIQ discrepancy, 74–76, 79, 80
relationships with WRAT scores,
76–78